"Mental health professionals hold key skills that can assist those living with inflammatory bowel disease from an emotional and physical perspective. This is an essential reading for those who would like to learn more about this disease and how to effectively contribute to integrative treatment planning utilizing evidence-based brain-gut psychological interventions. This manual will aid in increasing access to essential psychological treatment for those living life with IBD!"

Megan E. Riehl, *PsyD, AGAF, GI, Psychologist at the University of Michigan, USA, and Co-Author of* Mind Your Gut: The Science-Based, Whole-Body Guide to Living Well with IBS

"Cognitive behavioral therapy is the best researched psychological approach to support people living with IBD, but people with Crohn's and colitis often complain that their psychologists don't understand the challenges of living with these illnesses. The CBT program in this manual is easy to understand and apply in practice. Importantly, it explains IBD and its intricacies using a language accessible to non-medics. Case studies, in particular, show how to apply the CBT principles to real and complex life scenarios and how versatile and flexible CBT can be, making it easy to personalize for individual patients.

Dr. Hunt's book is a must read for any gastro-psychologist or mental health practitioner who supports people living with IBD, but also for physicians interested in going beyond treating the inflamed gut. The future of IBD care is biopsychosocial, with psychology a key element to helping our patients achieve optimal well-being. Dr. Melissa Hunt's book makes CBT for IBD easy."

Antonina Mikocka-Walus, *MA(Psych), PhD, Professor of Health Psychology and Leader of Mind-Body Research in Health Laboratory (MiRth), School of Psychology, Deakin University, Melbourne, Australia, and Co-Editor of* Psychogastroenterology for Adults: A Handbook for Mental Health Professionals

CBT for Patients with Inflammatory Bowel Disease

This treatment manual provides cognitive behavioral therapists with the inflammatory bowel disease (IBD) specific knowledge and content they need to work with this patient population.

Understanding the very real challenges of living with an IBD, and what sorts of catastrophic thoughts and maladaptive avoidance behaviors patients might have, can make therapy more focused, efficient, and effective. This manual encourages flexible, modular deployment of numerous empirically supported principles, techniques, and interventions, and includes five treatment protocols with hypothetical patients.

This book is essential for therapists with training in cognitive behavioral therapy who are interested in expanding their practice competence to work with patients with GI disorders, including inflammatory bowel disease.

Melissa G. Hunt is a licensed clinical psychologist and research scientist who specializes in helping folks with chronic GI disorders reclaim their lives. She serves as the Associate Director of Clinical Training in the Psychology Department at the University of Pennsylvania and is a member of the Rome Psychogastroenterology Group.

CBT for Patients with Inflammatory Bowel Disease

A Treatment Manual

MELISSA G. HUNT

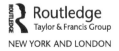
Routledge
Taylor & Francis Group

NEW YORK AND LONDON

Designed cover image: © Getty Images

First published 2024
by Routledge
605 Third Avenue, New York, NY 10158

and by Routledge
4 Park Square, Milton Park, Abingdon, Oxon, OX14 4RN

Routledge is an imprint of the Taylor & Francis Group, an informa business

ISBN: 978-1-032-59368-5 (hbk)
ISBN: 978-1-032-59360-9 (pbk)
ISBN: 978-1-003-45438-0 (ebk)

DOI: 10.4324/9781003454380

Typeset in Dante and Avenir
by Newgen Publishing UK

Dedicated *in memoriam* to

Dr. Dianne Chambless
1948–2023

I had the extraordinary privilege of counting Dianne as a colleague, mentor, and friend. Even after her retirement, I reached out to her often for advice and professional guidance, knowing that I would receive a wise and thoughtful return email usually within just a few hours. When I was considering my next professional challenge, she gently urged me to consider writing a treatment manual. One of my last email exchanges with her before her untimely death was to let her know that this very manual had been accepted for publication. She wrote back right away to tell me she was proud of me.

I hope she knew how much that meant to me.

Contents

About the Author

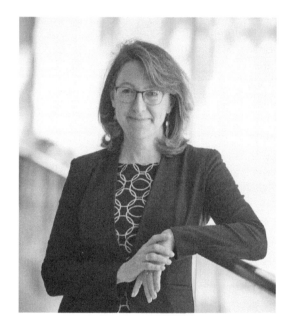

My name is Melissa G. Hunt and I'm a licensed clinical psychologist who specializes in cognitive behavioral therapy (CBT). I serve as the Associate Director of Clinical Training in the Department of Psychology at the University of Pennsylvania. I am very fortunate to be able to combine teaching, supervising young clinicians, doing research, and seeing patients. Like most clinical scientists, I find that each aspect of my professional life informs the others. I know that seeing patients makes me a better scientist, and doing research makes me a more effective therapist. I am always amazed that distressed people entrust me with their personal stories and are willing to share their pain in hopes that they may be able to feel better and to live richer, more productive, and more joyful lives. I've dedicated my career to using clinical science to advance well-being, and I am always thrilled when basic and applied science can be brought to bear to improve our treatments and to alleviate suffering.

Foreword

In the expansive landscape of health care, where our focus often gravitates toward clinical treatments and technological marvels, it's essential to recognize the profound influence of psychosocial factors on the well-being and function of individuals grappling with inflammatory bowel diseases (IBD).

IBD presents unique challenges to both physical and emotional health. The day to day experiences and mental well-being of individuals living with this condition are profoundly shaped by external factors that extend beyond the clinic or hospital walls. Amid the multifaceted challenges posed by IBD, mental health emerges as a vital aspect in need of our utmost attention—a facet intricately linked to how patients perceive and process their disease, the symptoms, treatment options (risks, benefits, and alternatives), and their relationship with their medical providers. These factors wield substantial influence over an individual's gastrointestinal symptoms, disease management, functional ability, and overall quality of life.

In this treatment manual explicating the use of cognitive behavioral therapy for adults with IBD, Dr. Hunt delves into the complex dynamics and relationships that shape the experiences of individuals facing this chronic disease. Dr. Hunt offers clinically effective interventions along with illustrative patient vignettes to actively address knowledge gaps and offers solutions, with the ultimate goal of enhancing the mental well-being of those living with IBD and reducing disability in IBD.

It is my hope that through this book, more behavioral health specialists will learn to work with this population. By training more GI-informed providers we can profoundly enhance the mental well-being and the overall quality of life and function of individuals navigating the challenging terrain of IBD.

—Dr. Chung Sang Tse, 2023
Assistant Professor of Clinical Medicine
Gastroenterology
University of Pennsylvania School of Medicine

Introduction

This manual provides a guide for therapists experienced with cognitive behavioral therapy (CBT) who would like to work with patients who have inflammatory bowel diseases (IBD). IBD include predominantly Crohn's disease and ulcerative colitis, and several other variants such as ulcerative proctitis, and indeterminate colitis. While IBD are biological immune-mediated diseases, psychotherapy with a knowledgeable CBT therapist can have a number of beneficial outcomes, including improved health related quality of life (HRQL), decreased distress and disability, decreased risk of comorbid depression and anxiety disorders, decreased risk of secondary irritable bowel syndrome (IBS), and even lower rates of relapse and better response to IBD specific medications. This treatment manual assumes good working knowledge of a number of core CBT principles and techniques for the treatment of depression, panic disorder and agoraphobia, health anxiety, social anxiety, obsessive-compulsive disorder, and post-traumatic stress disorder. It demonstrates how to apply a number of transdiagnostic techniques to this unique population, including relaxation training, deep diaphragmatic breathing, behavioral activation, thought records, cognitive reappraisal, de-catastrophizing, motivational interviewing, imaginal and *in vivo* exposure therapy, behavioral experiments, and mindfulness. These are all empirically supported, CBT interventions which can be mixed and matched depending on the individual patient's exact presentation and treatment goals.

The manual provides IBD specific knowledge and content that will often be the focus of sessions with people with IBD. For individuals with IBD, not having to explain the complexities of their disease and its management, and

DOI: 10.4324/9781003454380-1

not having to worry about embarrassing themselves or disgusting their therapist with references to diarrhea and other bodily processes and waste, is an incredible relief. For the therapist, knowing in advance both what the very real challenges of living with an IBD can be, *and* what sorts of catastrophic thoughts and maladaptive avoidance behaviors IBD patients might be likely to engage in can make the therapy much more focused, efficient, and effective.

The first part of the manual is intended to educate CBT therapists about IBD. The second part of the manual is the actual treatment guide, although it is not a traditional treatment manual with exact outlines of session by session content. Rather, the treatment guidelines are designed as modular skills which can be mixed and matched by the therapist depending on the needs of the individual patient. In all the modules, IBD-specific content is applied to either improving overall health related quality of life or to the treatment of a specific comorbid psychiatric diagnosis. In other words, the text encourages flexible deployment of numerous empirically supported principles and transdiagnostic techniques and interventions, with a good understanding of how the IBD may be central to the person's distress. The third part of the manual consists of five different patient case histories demonstrating the range of difficulties patients with IBD may have, and what a course of treatment might look like for patients with varying degrees of IBD severity, distress, disability, psychiatric comorbidity, and other psychosocial complexities.

If you don't think you can talk about anatomy, bodily processes, and waste with patients without embarrassment or disgust, or if you "don't want to know" those kinds of things about the patients you work with, then working with patients with IBD is not for you. That said, most CBT therapists have been trained to work with vomit and blood phobias, and with obsessive-compulsive disorder (OCD), which often involves exposure therapy to body fluids of all sorts, including sweat, vomit, blood, spit, mucus, urine, semen, and poop (or at least fake versions of them!). If you have experience with any of that, then it should be fairly easy for you to extend that basic training to this work. Very rarely will you or the patient need to engage in exposure therapy with actual bodily wastes. Rather, you need to provide a safe, disgust-free zone for patients to freely *talk* about their issues and concerns with someone who understands the ins and outs of living with an IBD. Just that can be therapeutic in and of itself.

Part I

Introduction to Inflammatory Bowel Diseases

What the Clinician Needs to Know

What are Inflammatory Bowel Diseases?   **1**

Types of IBD

Inflammatory bowel disease (IBD) is the collective term for a group of related, immune-mediated disorders in which the immune system mistakenly attacks healthy tissue in the digestive tract, and occasionally elsewhere in the body as well. The chronic inflammation causes damage to the digestive tract, which can result in ulcers, thickened scar tissue, obstructions, tears or perforations, fistulas (abnormal connections between the gut and other body parts), bleeding, malnutrition, weight loss, and an increased risk for cancer. There are several different types of IBD, predominantly including Crohn's disease and ulcerative colitis. Less common forms of IBD are ulcerative proctitis (ulcerative colitis that affects the rectum and anus only, i.e., the last 10–15 cm of the colon), indeterminate colitis (has features that could be either Crohn's disease or ulcerative colitis), and possibly microscopic colitis (though whether this is an IBD or a separate disease entirely is currently under debate). IBD are also associated with other immune-mediated diseases including rheumatoid arthritis and psoriasis, which can cause disability and distress themselves and concomitantly with IBD.

Crohn's disease is a subtype of IBD that can impact any part of the digestive tract. Although it mostly affects the intestines, it can also have extra-intestinal manifestations such as skin lesions, joint pain, and extreme fatigue. The most common symptoms of Crohn's disease are abdominal pain, frequent, urgent diarrhea, occasional constipation, bloody stools and, often, nutritional deficiencies, especially iron deficiency anemia and B12 deficiency, both of which

DOI: 10.4324/9781003454380-3

can cause significant fatigue and brain fog. People with flaring Crohn's disease may also experience mouth lesions, skin lesions, and joint pain.

Ulcerative colitis (UC) is the other main IBD and is also an immune-mediated disorder. UC, like Crohn's disease, can cause inflammation and ulcers in the lining of the rectum and colon, but unlike Crohn's disease the inflammation is typically limited to the large intestine. However, this doesn't make UC less serious. Ulcers can form where inflammation has damaged or killed the cells that usually line the colon. Similar to Crohn's disease, this can result in intestinal bleeding, leading to bloody stools and anemia. The most common symptoms of UC are burning or stabbing abdominal pain, cramps, and frequent, urgent diarrhea which may be watery, bloody, or full of mucus.

Ulcerative proctitis is a slightly less severe form of UC in which the inflammation is confined to the mucosa of the rectum and the tissues of the anus. It can cause lower abdominal pain, urgency, and passing blood or mucus from the rectum on its own or mixed with stool.

Microscopic colitis (MC) has historically been considered a variant of IBD in which the inflammatory changes are subtle and can only be seen under a microscope (but colonoscopy images of the gut appear normal). There is some debate about whether MC is a true IBD, or some other disease category, but MC is also thought to be an autoimmune disorder. Despite the subtlety of the changes, microscopic colitis can cause significant distress and disability in response to having persistent, watery, and often urgent diarrhea. Many people with MC also have other autoimmune problems which might include rheumatoid arthritis, psoriasis, celiac disease, or endocrine problems like Hashimoto's thyroiditis or Graves' disease. A history of having taken certain medications is known to increase the risk for MC. In particular, long term or chronic use of non-steroidal anti-inflammatory painkillers, including aspirin, ibuprofen (Motrin), and naproxen (Aleve), turns out to be very common in people who are ultimately diagnosed with MC. It might seem ironic that using an anti-inflammatory drug would increase the risk of an inflammatory bowel disorder. Unfortunately, this particular class of drugs tends to irritate the lining of the intestines.

Indeterminate colitis involves a minority of patients (around 5%), and this can be a frustrating diagnosis for them. It is typically given when a more definitive diagnosis of either Crohn's disease or UC cannot be made on the basis of colonoscopy or colonic biopsy. That is, the patient's colonoscopy has features that could be consistent with either Crohn's disease or UC. Despite the frustration and confusion that patients often experience when their doctor can't tell them *exactly* what they have, the treatments for indeterminate colitis are the same as they are for Crohn's disease and UC.

All the subtypes of IBD have a good deal of symptom overlap with irritable bowel syndrome (IBS). In fact, many patients with IBD are first mistakenly diagnosed with IBS, to their great frustration. IBS is a disorder of central-enteric pain processing, or gut-brain interaction, in which the brain starts to over-interpret signals from the gut and people develop visceral hypersensitivity. This leads to a positive feedback loop of increasing discomfort, anxiety, hypervigilance, catastrophizing, and stress, all of which in turn increase discomfort and urgency. The primary symptoms of IBS are frequent abdominal pain (at least once a week) and altered bowel habits, including predominant diarrhea (which can be urgent), predominant constipation, or an alternating mix of the two. IBS is *not* driven by inflammation and does *not* result in any tissue damage, and all the tests typically ordered by a gastroenterologist will come back negative or "normal." A number of studies have suggested that it is very difficult to distinguish IBS and microscopic colitis on the basis of symptom presentation alone. Indeed, many patients with histologically proven microscopic colitis will also technically meet diagnostic criteria for IBS. It is also important to note that people with definitively diagnosed IBD can also develop *secondary* IBS, and may still be symptomatic as a result even when their IBD is in remission.

What Complications Can Arise for IBD Patients?

Understanding the kinds of complications and crises IBD patients are sometimes faced with is important when working with them. While they can and sometimes do experience health anxiety and catastrophizing, they are also vulnerable to serious medical complications, some of which can be life threatening. Advocating for patients, encouraging them to reach out to their physicians when something feels wrong, and being able to empathize appropriately with the very real challenges of living with an IBD can all go a long way in delivering effective psychosocial treatment and support.

Urgency, Frequency, and Incontinence

Urgency and frequent bowel movements are probably the most common aspects of IBD that patients need to adjust to. It is not uncommon for a patient with even relatively well managed IBD to need to defecate (or poop) three to five times a day, and people with flaring IBD may poop even more frequently. Other patients will spend hours on the toilet every morning to try to "empty out" before heading out for the day in an attempt to forestall the inconvenience and potential embarrassment of needing to poop while out and about in public. As we will see in later sections on social anxiety and agoraphobia, fecal urgency, and worrying about fecal incontinence (FI) can cause significant distress and disability in patients with IBD. This is not just a catastrophic cognition or a distortion. Around 25% of patients with IBD have actually experienced at least one lifetime episode of FI. The likelihood of FI is associated with age, disease severity, and disease chronicity, but lots of relatively young patients with IBD still worry about it a lot, and may have had several "close calls" or a true episode of FI.

One useful tool for talking about poop with patients is the Bristol Stool Scale. It is a standard, seven point scale that describes the shape and consistency of stool. Most patients have heard about it from their doctor, and it can provide a convenient short-hand when discussing urgency (or constipation for that matter). It is easy to find charts of the Bristol Stool Scale online, complete with pictures representing each category of poop, but a basic description of the categories is below.

1–Separate, small, hard, dry pellets—"rabbit poop" as many patients call it. These are often associated with constipation and may be quite difficult to pass.
2–Hard, sausage-shaped, lumpy poop. This may also be difficult to pass and patients sometimes have to strain to move these out.
3–Coherent discrete sausage shapes that are softer than 2, but may still have cracks and texture on the surface.
4–Smooth, soft, long sausages or snakes.
5–Soft, separate blobs with clear cut edges. These sometimes come out in long very skinny pieces—"worms" or "pasta" poops as some patients refer to them.
6–Fluffy, mushy poop that coheres, but has no recognizable pieces or edges. Like a pile of wet souffle or pudding. It may also have recognizable bits of undigested food mixed in.
7–Entirely liquid and watery. No solid pieces or form whatsoever.

Many patients with IBD will note that the first bowel movement of the morning might be nicely formed—say a 4 or even a 3, but the next one of the morning 15 minutes later will be a 5, the next a 6 and finally they might have several rounds of liquid stool before feeling empty.

Weight Loss and Nutritional Deficiencies

Weight loss and nutritional deficiencies are common complications of IBD and may be the first symptoms that bring patients to the attention of a gastro-enterologist. Nutritional deficiencies are common, even when weight loss is not extreme, because an inflamed small intestine cannot absorb nutrients from food. Iron deficiency anemia and B12 deficiency are particularly common. Many IBD patients will need occasional iron infusions or B12 injections to maintain healthy levels of those nutrients. If your patient looks very pale, or is complaining of constant fatigue and brain fog, you should encourage them to talk to their doctor about getting blood work done to check their iron and B12 levels. Clinical "pallor" or paleness secondary to anemia can be harder to detect in dark-skinned people. Looking at the palms of the hands, the beds of the nails, the gums, or the conjunctivae around the eyes will typically alert a clinician to the possibility of anemia in these folks. Nail beds should be a healthy "pink" even in very dark-skinned people. Very pale or white nail beds are a huge red flag. Folks with iron or B12 deficiency will typically start oral supplements, but it might make more sense to receive an iron infusion or B12 injection, since oral supplements are not always well absorbed. Oral iron can also be problematic because it can cause constipation, but iron infusions are a great alternative if the patient's insurance will approve it, although the patient will have to go to an infusion center to have it done. Liquid oral iron supplements (drops) can also be a good alternative to oral iron tablets (pedi-atric patients typically use the liquid drops). The liquid iron drops tend to be better tolerated than the oral tablets. It is also a good alternative to IV. B12 can be taken as a sublingual, quick dissolving oral pill, or given in an injection in the doctor's office. A B12 injection can be a quick fix that can dramatically improve the patient's fatigue and cognitive fog. Remember that you will be seeing your patient far more often (and for longer sessions) than their doctor does. Therapists often "catch" nutritional deficiencies, and getting them corrected will make your patient feel *much* better.

Osteoporosis

Active IBD can contribute to osteopenia (weakening bones) and osteoporosis (weak, brittle bones) in several different ways. Steroids, which are often used to treat IBD, can damage bone cells and impair the formation of new cells. They also reduce the absorption of calcium in the intestines, a mineral which is crucial for bone health. People taking systemic steroids are at higher risk of fractures. Fortunately, the risk of fracture tends to normalize when you stop taking steroids. Unfortunately, the IBD itself can also contribute to osteoporosis. Nutrient malabsorption from the IBD can also reduce available calcium, vitamin D, and vitamin K, all three of which are necessary for maintaining and replenishing bone strength. Finally, inflammatory cytokines which are common in IBD can impair new bone formation and can even cause bone resorption. Our bodies synthesize vitamin D from sunshine, but many people will be found to be vitamin D deficient on bloodwork. An interesting conundrum with dark-skinned people is that lower levels of vitamin D (specifically 25-hydroxyvitamin D, which is actually a precursor of the active vitamin) are very common in people of African descent (presumably because higher levels of melanin in the skin block the rays necessary for vitamin D production) but don't seem to be correlated with bone density issues to the same extent they are for lighter-skinned people. On the other hand, dark-skinned people often have normal levels of 1,25-dihydroxyvitamin D, which is the active metabolite, and in the general population, people of African descent are at relatively low risk of osteoporosis. So it isn't clear whether the standard blood test for vitamin D deficiency means the same thing for people of African descent. Nevertheless, vitamin D deficiency has been linked to greater risk of other problems in people of African descent, including diabetes, so supplementing with a modest dose of vitamin D is probably a good idea for most patients with IBD, regardless of skin color.

Obesity

Surprisingly, anywhere from 15–40% of adults with IBD will actually meet criteria for obesity, with another 10–20% being significantly overweight. This is partly because being overweight or obese to begin with puts people at higher risk of developing an IBD. But it is also because having an IBD can paradoxically lead to significant weight gain. First, people with IBD often rely on low fiber, "easy" to digest, highly processed foods like rice, pasta, white bread, and crackers, while avoiding foods high in insoluble fiber like whole grains, most vegetables, and many fruits. They sometimes load all their daily calories into a single meal (often at the end of the workday when they are back in the "safety" of their home), focusing on calorie dense foods that are not particularly healthful. Moreover, data suggest that dysbiosis and altered metabolic gut signaling induced by IBD can impact hormones, satiety related peptides, and bile acids, all of which can lead to metabolic changes and inadvertent weight gain. Many patients with IBD who used to smoke are motivated to successfully quit smoking, which is crucial for managing an inflammatory condition, but often results in significant weight gain. Finally, taking steroids often results in significant weight gain. It can be hard for patients who are struggling with eating and digestion to be told by nutritionists, physicians, or behavioral health therapists that they need to lose weight. But obesity itself can contribute to worsening inflammation throughout the body, and can make intervening effectively for IBD (especially with surgery) much more difficult and more likely to result in complications. It can also be difficult for patients with IBD to have their concerns about getting enough nutrition taken seriously when they are visibly overweight.

Constipation and Pelvic Floor Dysfunction

One ironic complication of IBD may be chronic constipation. Some patients develop pelvic floor dysfunction from years of trying to "hold in" diarrhea. This can result in overly tight, constricted muscles in the anal sphincter and pelvic floor resulting in difficulty with defecation. The muscles contract abnormally or may have difficulty sensing the presence or absence of stool in the rectum. Defecatory dyssynergia, in which the muscles of the rectum and the anal sphincter don't work in concert with each other, can cause constipation. The rectum may squeeze, but if the anal sphincter remains tightly closed, the stool cannot exit. Left unmanaged, chronic constipation and stool retention can cause problems of their own, including hemorrhoids (both external and internal, which can bleed, which is alarming, and can be quite itchy and uncomfortable) and descending perineum syndrome (where the tissues of the pelvic floor between the front of the pelvis and the anus bulge out during defecation),typically as a result of frequent straining. Many of these pelvic floor issues can be addressed with pelvic floor physical therapy, and it may fall to the therapist to suggest this to a patient and encourage them to follow through on it. Pelvic floor physical therapists are wonderful people—kind, discreet, empathetic, and often able to use humor to coach patients through otherwise embarrassing or awkward procedures.

Strictures

Many folks with an IBD will develop scar tissue in the gut as ulcers heal. Because scar tissue is often thick, rigid, and tight, IBD patients can develop *strictures* or points where the intestinal tube becomes quite narrow or constricted. When a tube is narrow, things move through it more slowly. Thus, while watery diarrhea is a common symptom of IBD, some IBD patients will actually also experience slowed motility (the contractions of the gut that move waste through) and increased transit time (the time it takes for food to work its way through from the mouth to the anus). When the tube is very narrow, food waste can get backed up behind it and goes through very slowly—like a highway narrowing from four lanes down to one. Waste gets through, but not as quickly as it should. This can lead to high stool load further up from the stricture, which can cause considerable discomfort, bloating, and gas buildup. It can also result in constipation and infrequent bowel movements that may be hard and dry and difficult or even painful to pass. This is another reason many patients with IBD prefer to avoid high fiber foods, fruits, and vegetables.

Bowel Obstructions

In the most dangerous variant of this, IBD patients may experience a *bowel obstruction* which can occur either in the colon (less common) or in the small intestine (small bowel obstruction or SBO) in which food waste gets trapped at a point of stricture. Bowel obstructions can be partial (some food waste is stuck but material can pass around it) or complete (no gas or stool can pass) and are typically quite painful. In an SBO, waste and water can end up backing up into the stomach, causing nausea and vomiting. The abdomen often becomes distended and bloated with trapped gas and stool. With a complete obstruction, people will be unable to pass gas or to have a bowel movement, resulting in total constipation and severe cramping. Bowel obstructions *can* resolve on their own, but if they fail to resolve within a few hours, the patient should head into the ER. Untreated, a bowel obstruction can be life threatening. In the hospital, staff will conduct imaging to confirm the obstruction, and will keep the patient on IV fluids with nothing to eat until the obstruction resolves. They might also decompress the bowel with a naso-gastric tube. In the most extreme cases, surgery may be necessary. If surgery is required, but diagnosis is delayed by more than 36 hours, the mortality rate can be as high as 10%. Thus, patients need to understand the symptoms of an SBO, and know when to get emergency medical care.

This is why many gastroenterologists encourage patients with IBD who have strictures to avoid specific *high residue foods* that are chunky, stringy, or sharp and are more likely to get stuck. This includes popcorn, corn chips, celery, whole nuts and seeds and dried fruits. Young adult patients may get frustrated with these limitations (who doesn't want to be able to eat chips and salsa at the bar or have popcorn at the movies with their friends?) and may need help to "make peace" with these dietary restrictions. On the other hand, an older IBD patient who has experienced an SBO and/or had surgery, may sometimes develop an unnecessarily restricted diet—for example eating only pureed baby food—in order to prevent a possible future SBO. These folks may need help overcoming their (understandable) anxiety about the impact of food and may need to undertake some exposure therapy to broaden their diet.

Fistulas

Fistulas are another potential complication of IBD. Fistulas are small tubes that form when an ulcer goes all the way through the intestinal wall, creating a connection to some other part of the body. Fistulas can form between two different parts of the intestine, or between the small and large intestine. They can also form between the intestine and the skin, bladder, or (in women) between the rectum and the vagina. Where fistulas are present, food waste and bacteria can pass out of the intestine into the other body parts or through to the skin, increasing the risk of infection. Fistulas that form between the intestine and the skin, where they usually present as a painful bump or boil, can open up causing an abscess to form which may drain pus or even stool. In a rectal–vaginal fistula, the vagina may leak stool uncontrollably, which is messy, and raises the risk of vaginal infections dramatically. Many women with a rectal–vaginal fistula are afraid that others will smell the stool and will find them disgusting. At its best, it is a lot to manage and requires creative and flexible problem solving and *lots* of extra hygiene. If a female patient tells you that she has a fistula, be sure to ask *where it is*. If it involves the vagina, be sure to empathize and ask her how she is managing it. Fistulas of any kind can be painful, embarrassing, and even dangerous. They are typically treated with medication, but may require surgical correction. Fistulas are becoming slightly less common as medications for IBD improve, but about 30% of Crohn's patients may develop one at some point. They are slightly less common for UC patients, but are still possible. Having a therapist who understands what a fistula is and is willing to talk about it and brainstorm how to manage it can be a huge relief for IBD patients.

Cancer

One of the scariest complications of IBD is cancer. IBD puts patients at increased risk of colon cancer, and that is often one of the top concerns patients have. Cancer surveillance is one of the reasons that GI guidelines for IBD management include repeat colonoscopies every one to two years. This can be tough on patients (no one enjoys colonoscopies) but it can be lifesaving. Many medications that are used to treat IBD ironically have *different* cancers (especially skin cancer and lymphoma) as potential adverse effects. It is important to remind patients that while taking those medications might increase their risk of getting cancer, *not* treating their IBD *also* increases their cancer risk.

Irritable Bowel Syndrome

The final "complication" of IBD isn't really a complication at all as much as a frequent comorbidity. Recall that many patients with IBD are initially *mis*diagnosed with IBS. So it can be truly confusing to patients to hear that they have developed secondary IBS even when their IBD is in medical remission. Unfortunately, this is all too common. About 35% of patients whose IBD is in long standing remission will still experience significant GI symptoms consistent with IBS, including frequent abdominal pain, diarrhea, constipation or an alternating mix of the two, gas, bloating, and urgency. The overall population prevalence of IBS is anywhere between 6% and 15%, so IBD constitutes a significant risk factor for developing IBS. Both patients and their doctors may be very frustrated by this. Pathology results from biopsies may even confirm remission at the histologic (or cellular) level, but the patient is still symptomatic, and is still experiencing considerable distress and disability. These patients report significantly lower health related quality of life than patients without secondary IBS.

Fortunately, IBS is very amenable to treatment from a cognitive behavioral perspective. It also responds well to GI directed hypnotherapy. Mindfulness based interventions can also be helpful. Basically, the goal is to retrain the brain to stop amplifying and worrying about the signals from the gut. Of course, patients with IBD sometimes NEED to pay attention to GI discomfort and symptoms. Abdominal pain could indicate active flares or even bowel obstructions. Diarrhea and urgency could suggest that their medication isn't working well anymore. It can be tricky to tease apart the GI discomfort of IBS from the GI discomfort of escalating IBD. But most patients will tell you that, once they start paying attention, they realize that the pain of IBS is different from the pain of IBD. If your patient has developed secondary IBS in the context of medically stable IBD, focus your work on helping the patient to not catastrophize the discomfort. Refocus on deep diaphragmatic breathing and mindful attention training exercises. Ensure that they are not falling back on agoraphobic avoidance. Patients are often surprised by how quickly the pain and urgency recede. CBT practices can definitely help patients learn to *cope* with the GI discomfort of IBD, but CBT practices can actually dramatically *reduce* the GI discomfort of IBS. So helping patients learn to distinguish between the two can be enormously helpful.

Summary

Inflammatory bowel diseases are serious biological, immune-mediated disorders that can have potentially life-threatening complications. Having a therapist who understands at least these basic aspects of the disease can be a huge relief for patients. They don't have to justify and *explain* why their abdominal pain the night before was so scary (because they have a history of transient small bowel obstructions). They know you'll get why they are so frustrated that their insurance won't authorize the capsule endoscopy, forcing them to endure the full prep for a colonoscopy instead. They can give you their medical history and talk about bloody poop and urgency and stained underwear without embarrassment or shame. I like to tell patients up front that I have no disgust sensitivity about these issues, and they should feel free to be as graphic and specific as they like. I've heard it all, and nothing about it will bother me. Just having a safe space to talk about all this with someone who is objective, but knowledgeable, understanding, and empathetic is often highly therapeutic in and of itself.

Bibliography

Ballou, S. & Keefer, L. (2017). Psychological interventions for irritable bowel syndrome and inflammatory bowel diseases. *Clinical and Translational Gastroenterology*, 8(1), e214.

Berg, D. F., Bahadursingh, A. M., Kaminski, D. L. & Longo, W. E. (2002). Acute surgical emergencies in inflammatory bowel disease. *The American Journal of Surgery,* *184*(1), 45–51.

Büsch, K., Sonnenberg, A. & Bansback, N. (2014). Impact of inflammatory bowel disease on disability. *Current Gastroenterology Reports, 16,* 1–9.

Chang, J. T. (2020). Pathophysiology of inflammatory bowel diseases. *New England Journal of Medicine, 383*(27), 2652–2664.

Chumpitazi, B. P., Self, M. M., Czyzewski, D. I., Cejka, S., Swank, P. R. & Shulman, R. J. (2016). Bristol Stool Form Scale reliability and agreement decreases when determining Rome III stool form designations. *Neurogastroenterology & Motility,* *28*(3), 443–8.

Fairbrass, K. M., Costantino, S. J., Gracie, D. J. & Ford, A. C. (2020). Prevalence of irritable bowel syndrome-type symptoms in patients with inflammatory bowel disease in remission: a systematic review and meta-analysis. *The Lancet Gastroenterology &* *Hepatology, 5*(12), 1053–1062.

Gu, P., Kuenzig, M. E., Kaplan, G. G., Pimentel, M. & Rezaie, A. (2018). Fecal incontinence in inflammatory bowel disease: a systematic review and meta-analysis. *Inflammatory Bowel Diseases, 24*(6), 1280–1290.

Kotze, P. G., Shen, B., Lightner, A., Yamamoto, T., Spinelli, A., Ghosh, S. & Panaccione, R. (2018). Modern management of perianal fistulas in Crohn's disease: future directions. *Gut, 67*(6), 1181–1194.

Norton, C., Dibley, L. B. & Bassett, P. (2013). Faecal incontinence in inflammatory bowel disease: associations and effect on quality of life. *Journal of Crohn's and Colitis, 7*(8), e302–e311.

Ramos, G. P. & Papadakis, K. A. (2019). Mechanisms of disease: inflammatory bowel diseases. *Mayo Clinic Proceedings,* (94)1,155–165).

Rubin, D. C., Shaker, A. & Levin, M. S. (2012). Chronic intestinal inflammation: inflammatory bowel disease and colitis-associated colon cancer. *Frontiers in Immunology, 3,* 107.

Shah, N. D. (2015). Low residue vs. low fiber diets in inflammatory bowel disease: evidence to support vs. habit? *Practical Gastroenterology, 39*(7), 48–57.

How are IBD Diagnosed?

2

The Journey to Diagnosis

Historically, for most people who were ultimately diagnosed with an inflammatory bowel disease, the journey to diagnosis was long and harrowing. Many older patients have been through the proverbial medical wringer—seeing an average of five different doctors, undergoing an average of eight to nine diagnostic tests, and spending more than a year feeling very ill (with almost half having been hospitalized at least once) before they finally got a confirmatory diagnosis. Younger patients today have typically been diagnosed more quickly, but they may still have experienced anywhere from three months to a full year of uncertainty, dismissive doctors or ER staff, and anxiety, not to mention that it's even less fun for a 15 year old to need a colonoscopy than it is for a 50 year old. (Today, the median time to diagnosis for Crohn's is eight months, and for UC it's about four months.) Delayed diagnosis is associated with disease progression, higher odds of developing strictures and fistulas, and needing surgery, so it's a good thing that median times to diagnosis have decreased.

It's important for a therapist to understand the various diagnostic procedures that are used to confirm (or rule out) IBD and can also be used to track disease severity, medication response, and monitor for disease complications. Many patients may themselves be confused or ambivalent about undergoing these procedures, interpreting the results, or understanding the implications of the test results. While the patient should obviously rely on their gastroenterologist,

DOI: 10.4324/9781003454380-4

the therapist can often play a helpful role in addressing fear or reluctance, normalizing the procedures and helping patients think through the various treatment options that have been presented to them.

Blood and Stool Tests

Most patients will present to a gastroenterologist initially with complaints of frequent abdominal pain, diarrhea, and sometimes constipation and/or weight loss and fatigue. The GI doctor will usually order blood work and stool tests first. Using blood tests, they will check the complete blood count (CBC), sedimentation rate, and C-reactive protein, all of which might reveal underlying inflammation. They should also check the hemoglobin, ferritin, and vitamin B12 levels. Many people with an active IBD will show signs of anemia, which can suggest that ulcers in the intestines are causing bleeding and/or that they are not absorbing sufficient iron from their food. B12 deficiencies are also common in Crohn's because B12 is absorbed by the ileum (the last section of the small intestine) which is a very common location for Crohn's inflammation. In addition to blood work, the doctor should also ask the patient to collect small stool sample smears for several days, and will check those samples for blood (called a fecal occult blood test), which can also suggest bleeding in the intestines.

A savvy doctor will also order a specific stool test called the *fecal calprotectin test*. This is a non-invasive test that requires a fair bit of stool, which the patient must collect in a plastic bucket-like insert for the toilet and then scoop into the sample container and return to the lab. The stool is then tested for an inflammatory marker that is associated with IBD. The fecal calprotectin test is both fairly sensitive and quite specific to IBD, although it can miss Crohn's disease that is active only in the small intestine. Unfortunately, some GI doctors don't routinely run this test, which is one reason that some IBD patients are misdiagnosed with IBS early on. Doctors should also run blood work to check for celiac disease, a different autoimmune disorder in which the immune system reacts to gluten, the protein in wheat, and attacks the cilia of the small intestine. Patients must continue eating gluten-containing foods for about six weeks prior to the test so that the celiac specific antibodies will be present in the blood if the person does indeed have celiac disease. Note that folks with IBD are actually at higher risk for celiac disease than the general population and may suffer from both disorders.

Scopes

If any of the blood or stool markers come back suspicious for inflammation, or if there is blood in the stool, the GI doctor will almost certainly want to do a colonoscopy or sigmoidoscopy. In both a sigmoidoscopy and a colonoscopy, the doctor inserts a flexible lighted tube into the anus and up through part of the large intestine. Flexible sigmoidoscopy lets the doctor see only the last third of the large intestine (the sigmoid colon). Colonoscopy allows the doctor to see the *entire* large intestine, and *sometimes* the terminal ileum (or the last bit of the small intestine) so it's usually the better procedure, although it does take a bit more time and effort to prepare for it. In both cases, the scope transmits images of the lining of the intestine to a computer or video monitor. The doctor can actually *see* if there is any inflammation, ulceration, or bleeding. Both procedures also allow the doctor to remove any polyps or other growths and to take very small samples of tissue or biopsies, which can then be looked at carefully under a microscope. The pathology report will then report on the histology (microanatomy of the cells taken during the biopsies) to confirm whether or not an inflammatory process is at work. This is what is referred to as "histological confirmation of the diagnosis."

For the vast majority of people, the worst part of a "scope" is the prep the day before. The bowel needs to be cleaned out of all food waste and stool. This means the person has to take large quantities of stool softener and laxatives and consume nothing but liquids the day before the test. Very unfortunately, recent instructions from many GI practices are to start the "clean out" late in the day—around 4 or 5 pm. This is so that the person could, in theory, work during the day of the prep, even though they can't eat anything besides clear liquids. I strongly recommend to my patients that they take the entire day off and start the prep earlier in the day. If you start in the early evening, many people will be up pretty much all night on and off the toilet with urgent or even uncontrollable diarrhea. This is exhausting and unnecessary. Far better to schedule the procedure first thing in the morning if possible, and take off from work to start the prep mid-morning the day before.

On the other hand, some patients with IBD are so used to having urgent, watery diarrhea that the scope prep doesn't bother them that much. That should give you a sense of what some of these folks are living with every day.

The procedure itself is almost always done under anesthesia, usually with a very short acting agent like propofol. Most people wake up very quickly and throw off the grogginess easily. Very few people report feeling "drugged" or nauseous after the procedure. Rather, most people just feel somewhat lightheaded (from hunger) and are eager to get something to eat when they get home. Unfortunately, the GI doctor will often come to the patient's bedside shortly after they wake up to give them the first set of results (what they were able to see and how many polyps they might have removed). People often have trouble encoding and remembering what the doctor says, and will need to confirm what they heard later on, perhaps by viewing the results in a patient portal. The final results come after any biopsies have been evaluated by the pathology lab, and may not be available for one to two weeks.

Imaging

There are a number of other diagnostic tests or imaging procedures that a GI doctor may order, and it is important for a psychotherapist to review with a patient which procedures they have undergone and what the results were. It's very difficult for doctors to get physical scopes with cameras and biopsy tools into most of the small intestine, and it's important to get a look at it, since Crohn's disease activity is sometimes confined to the small intestine. Therefore, they will often order one or more imaging studies that will give them a sense of what's going on in the part of the intestines they can't directly access during a scope.

In an upper GI and small bowel series, or CT scan the patient will need to drink barium, a slightly sweet, chalky white liquid that coats the lining of the small intestine, making it easier to see what's going on. After drinking the barium, they will have x-rays or a CT scan taken. The barium looks white in the images, and shows spots where there may be inflammation or other abnormalities in the small intestine. While many doctors and hospitals still use these tried and true procedures, a newer way to visualize the intestines is with MRE (magnetic resonance enterography—which is really just an MRI of the gut). MRE is more sensitive to real time changes than CT scans are, so it's able to tell the difference between a narrowing that's due to normal peristalsis (muscle contractions that move food along) and a narrowing that's due to a stricture, or the formation of scar tissue. It also doesn't entail any radiation exposure, so it's safer than CT or barium x-ray, especially if the patient may need multiple scans throughout their life. Of course, it's also more expensive, so sometimes insurance won't cover it. If the patient is claustrophobic, or worried about a reaction to the contrast dye that must be injected, you may need to help them with CBT strategies to address panic, and you may need to encourage them to check with the doctor about any possible allergic reactions or contraindications for the dye.

The best way to visualize the entire small intestine is with a *capsule endoscopy*. In this amazing procedure, the patient swallows a tiny camera that is safely inside a capsule no bigger than a large vitamin pill. As it travels through the GI tract, it transmits multiple pictures to a small receiver worn on a belt. Many doctors will have the patient do a *patency test* first. In this procedure, the patient swallows a dissolvable dummy capsule the same size and shape as the camera capsule. The dummy capsule has a tiny tag inside it that can be identified by x-ray. If the capsule is still inside the body after 30 hours, this suggests that the real capsule might get stuck and would need to be retrieved surgically, generally making it not worth the risk. (People with chronic IBD may well have narrow spots in their intestines due to scar tissue or strictures, so the risk of the capsule getting stuck is real.) The dummy capsule will dissolve on its own and typically will not cause any problems. Assuming the patient passes the patency test, then they can proceed with the actual endoscopy. The camera capsule is disposable and passes out of the digestive system with a bowel movement. Patients need not physically retrieve the camera, but they do need to confirm that it has passed through them. The advantage of this procedure is that it lets the doctor see the *entire* small intestine. The disadvantage is that there's no way to take tissue samples, so there are no biopsies to analyze. But all of these procedures allow the doctor to actually *see* if there is any inflammation, ulcers, fistulas, strictures, or other signs of Crohn's in any part of the intestine.

Intestinal ultrasound (IUS) is an emerging technology that is fairly low cost (unlike MRE), safe (no radiation, nothing to swallow that might get stuck), well tolerated and convenient (no preparation), and appears to be highly sensitive and specific to IBD activity and complications. It has good accuracy in the diagnosis of both Crohn's and UC, and can be used to assess disease activity, the extent of involvement throughout the intestinal tract, and the presence of disease related complications including strictures, fistulas, and abscesses. It can also be used repeatedly to monitor response to therapy. IUS can be performed in a point-of-care setting (rather than a surgical center), leading to therapy optimization without delay, allowing repeated evaluations to monitor lesions over time, and even replacing invasive examinations, such as scopes. Unfortunately, as of this writing, it is only available at a few academic medical centers. However, more doctors are undertaking the necessary training and more centers are purchasing the ultrasound machines themselves, so we can hope that this diagnostic and disease monitoring technology will be more broadly available in years to come.

Even once a patient is diagnosed definitively, they may well have to undergo many of these diagnostic procedures repeatedly (every few years, yearly, or even more frequently) to track the state of their disease and monitor their response to medications. This can be time consuming and frustrating, but is an important aspect of medical management.

Summary

Patients with IBD must undergo a range of tests, some of which are fairly non-invasive (like blood work), some of which require handling and transporting various amounts of poop (like the fecal calprotectin test), some of which require visits to imaging centers to drink barium (for a CT scan) or to undergo an MRI with contrast dye, some of which require swallowing and wearing technology (a capsule endoscopy) and some of which require significant prep with laxatives and general anesthesia (like colonoscopies). Most patients will have to undergo various of these procedures multiple times in their life to monitor the disease, even if they are fairly medically stable. This can be burdensome, time consuming, expensive (depending on insurance coverage), and anxiety provoking. Intestinal ultrasound is an emerging technology that may spare patients some of the more invasive or risky procedures, but it is not available in many places just yet. Therapists can help patients think through the value of these procedures, and can help them overcome anxiety and avoidance, thus facilitating appropriate medical management of the disease. While it is ultimately the responsibility of the gastroenterologist to determine which tests to order and when they are necessary, therapists can help patients weigh the risks and benefits of each type so that patients are confident that they are making the best decisions possible in collaboration with their physician. Simply understanding the ins and outs of each of these procedures, helping patients plan the prep, and providing emotional support, care, and concern both before and after can be highly therapeutic, so don't shy away from talking about testing with patients.

Bibliography

Amitai, M. M., Ben-Horin, S., Eliakim, R. & Kopylov, U. (2013). Magnetic resonance enterography in Crohn's disease: a guide to common imaging manifestations for the IBD physician. *Journal of Crohn's and Colitis*, 7(8), 603–615.

Chang, S., Malter, L. & Hudesman, D. (2015). Disease monitoring in inflammatory bowel disease. *World Journal of Gastroenterology: WJG*, 21(40), 11246.

Flynn, S. & Eisenstein, S. (2019). Inflammatory bowel disease presentation and diagnosis. *Surgical Clinics*, 99(6), 1051–1062.

Fraquelli, M., Castiglione, F., Calabrese, E. & Maconi, G. (2020). Impact of intestinal ultrasound on the management of patients with inflammatory bowel disease: how to apply scientific evidence to clinical practice. *Digestive and Liver Disease*, 52(1), 9–18.

Gecse, K. B. & Vermeire, S. (2018). Differential diagnosis of inflammatory bowel disease: limitations and complications. *The Lancet Gastroenterology & Hepatology*, 3(9), 644–653.

Hosoe, N., Hayashi, Y. & Ogata, H. (2020). Colon capsule endoscopy for inflammatory bowel disease. *Clinical Endoscopy*, 53(5), 550–554.

Kaitha, S., Bashir, M. & Ali, T. (2015). Iron deficiency anemia in inflammatory bowel disease. *World Journal of Gastrointestinal Pathophysiology*, 6(3), 62.

Kopylov, U., Nemeth, A., Koulaouzidis, A., Makins, R., Wild, G., Afif, W., Bitton, A., Johansson, G. W., Bessissow, T., Eliakim, R., Toth, E. & Seidman, E. G. (2015). Small bowel capsule endoscopy in the management of established Crohn's disease: clinical impact, safety, and correlation with inflammatory biomarkers. *Inflammatory Bowel Diseases*, 21(1), 93–100.

Manetta, R., Capretti, I., Belleggia, N., Marsecano, C., Viscido, A., Bruno, F., Arrigoni, F., Ma, L., Guglielmi, G., Splendiani, A., Di Cesare, E., Masciocchi, C. & Barile, A. (2019). Magnetic resonance enterography (MRE) and ultrasonography (US) in the study of the small bowel in Crohn's disease: state of the art and review of the literature. *Acta Bio Medica: Atenei Parmensis*, 90(Suppl 5), 38.

Nemeth, A., Kopylov, U., Koulaouzidis, A., Johansson, G. W., Thorlacius, H., Amre, D., ... & Toth, E. (2016). Use of patency capsule in patients with established Crohn's disease. *Endoscopy*, 48(04), 373–379.

Tukey, M., Pleskow, D., Legnani, P., Cheifetz, A. S. & Moss, A. C. (2009). The utility of capsule endoscopy in patients with suspected Crohn's disease. *Official Journal of the American College of Gastroenterology| ACG*, 104(11), 2734–2739.

Walsham, N. E. & Sherwood, R. A. (2016). Fecal calprotectin in inflammatory bowel disease. *Clinical and Experimental Gastroenterology*, 21–29.

Ward, M. G., Kariyawasam, V. C., Mogan, S. B., Patel, K. V., Pantelidou, M., Sobczyńska-Malefora, A., ... & Irving, P. M. (2015). Prevalence and risk factors for functional vitamin B12 deficiency in patients with Crohn's disease. *Inflammatory Bowel Diseases*, 21(12), 2839–2847.

How are IBD Treated?   **3**

Many patients with IBD spend a good deal of time and energy thinking about the management of their disease. It can be important for the therapist to have a basic understanding about the types of dietary interventions, medications, and surgeries IBD patients may be treated with. Many people with IBD will need help and support in making decisions about whether or not to take a particular medication, whether to switch medications, or whether to heed their doctor's advice to consider surgery. While a therapist should always defer to the doctor's expertise, there is an important role for therapy in helping patients objectively weigh the potential costs and benefits of any particular approach, and in addressing their fears and frustrations. In particular, it is worth discussing the concept of omission error bias with patients. Like most human beings, people with IBD tend to focus more on the potential risks of *doing* something that ends up having a bad outcome (commission errors) than they do on the risks of *not* doing something and ending up with a bad outcome (omission error). Helping patients think through the risks and benefits of *both* choices is often helpful. For example, some IBD medications increase the risk of specific cancers, including lymphoma and skin cancer. That's true and it sucks. But untreated IBD itself *also* increases the risk of cancer, especially colon cancer. In fact, the risks of untreated IBD (including cancer, ongoing inflammation, serious complications) are statistically much higher than the risks involved in treatment. So patients need to weigh *both* risks and decide which one they can live with. People often forget that sometimes doing nothing entails *more* risk than doing something.

DOI: 10.4324/9781003454380-5

The Doctor/Patient/Therapist Relationship

As with most medical things, establishing a collaborative, respectful relationship with a highly skilled and caring doctor is one of the most important first steps a patient can take in managing an IBD. Unfortunately, many patients don't feel they have that. Sometimes it is because of a mismatch between patient preferences and the doctor's style. Some patients want detailed explanations of all test results and treatment options. They want to understand exactly what is going on in their body, and they want to be able to weigh the potential risks and benefits of various treatment approaches themselves. They will want a highly respectful relationship with a doctor who takes the time to educate them and takes their opinions and preferences seriously. This is often referred to as the collaborative care model. Other patients want a doctor who will make clear recommendations without burdening them with too much detailed information that might feel overwhelming and hard to understand. They don't want the responsibility of managing their own care or making complex medical decisions. After all, they didn't go to medical school—the doctor did! They want a kind, empathetic *expert* who will tell them what they would recommend if the patient were the doctor's own loved one. While the paternalistic, "doctor knows best" approach has fallen out of favor for good reason, the reality is that many patients appreciate it when the doctor/expert tells them what they think they should do. A third model is one in which the doctor attempts to find out what is most important to the patient. Do they want to minimize the risk of hospitalization or surgery? Do they want to feel better right away so they can enjoy life and meet their role obligations? Can they live with some abdominal pain and urgency for a while, but are terrified of the side effects of medications? A wise physician will devise a treatment plan that addresses the patient's values and concerns, while still giving evidence based treatment recommendations. A mismatch between doctor style and patient preference can make things much harder for both parties. You can strongly encourage your patients to be explicit with their doctor about what they prefer.

It is true that doctors are incredibly busy and have many demands on their time, and multiple streams of information they have to track all the time. But again, you should encourage your patient to make sure they get their questions answered and that their doctor responds to their concerns. It's a good idea for them to have a list of questions and concerns on paper (or in their phone) when they go to their appointment. This will help them

remember what they want to ask in a short amount of time and will provide some structure to the appointment. It can be hard to remember what
you wanted to talk about when you're being hit with recent test results or
new treatment options. But even the most well prepared patient will find that
things will inevitably come up in the appointment that the patient won't have
time or the focus to ask about further. Lots of hospitals have online patient
portal systems that let patients communicate securely with their doctor via
electronic messaging. Encourage them to take advantage of it.

If the patient feels that their doctor is being dismissive or rude, doesn't
have appropriate multicultural competence, or isn't taking their concerns seriously, the first thing to do is to encourage the patient to talk to their doctor
about it. The vast majority of doctors are truly decent, caring human beings
who want to provide compassionate care. They're just overwhelmed at times.
But if they try to talk to their doctor and they still feel uncomfortable or
unhappy with their care, it may be time to try to find a new doctor. This can
be hard outside of big cities with several major medical centers, but finding
a doctor the patient feels comfortable with, who respects them, takes plenty
of time, and answers their questions, is a really important part of managing
an IBD.

Of course, this works both ways! Part of collaborating effectively with a
doctor means that the patient also has to communicate in a clear and timely
way *with them*. If the patient has recently started a new medication, or has
undergone a diagnostic procedure, they should call their doctor as soon as
anything seems to be going wrong. Even if the side effects don't seem serious,
they should let their doctor make sure they aren't indicative of something
more concerning. Even if a patient has been on a particular medication for a
while, they should always let their doctor know if there is a change in their
symptoms or their experience. *The patient* is an incredibly important member
of their own treatment team. Many people hesitate to pick up the phone and
let their doctor know when something doesn't feel right. People often think to
themselves "I don't want to bother him or her or waste his or her time. I don't
want to be *that* patient that complains or is seen as whiny or bothersome or
wimpy." It's important to help patients understand that this drives doctors
crazy! No physician in their right mind would be bothered by a patient calling
in about a genuine alteration in symptoms or sensations. They *want* patients
to keep them informed in a timely way about the course of treatment. If the
patient doesn't call them, they are left in the dark and can't provide excellent
care, and that frustrates them more than anything. A problem that would be

minor if caught right away can become major if it's left unmanaged. Help patients understand that their doctor would MUCH rather hear from them right away than find out days later that a problem has escalated and is now going to be much more complicated to fix.

For patients, communicating effectively with a doctor also means being honest and transparent with them about a number of things, including embarrassing symptoms (like fecal incontinence or sexual issues) and issues related to taking medication as prescribed. Lots of patients forget to take their medicine at the right time. Or hesitate to take the full dose. Or fill the script but don't take the medication at all. Or don't follow up on getting lab work done or scheduling a necessary colonoscopy. Ask your patient if they've ever done any of these things, or if they're doing it now, and let them know that it's really important to be honest with their doctor about it. The doctor can't make reasonable decisions about whether a treatment is working if they don't know what the patient is actually doing. From a therapist's perspective, this is very similar to a patient informing you that they are not taking the medication prescribed by their psychiatrist. Your job is to help facilitate more honest and direct communication between the patient and the prescribing physician. Patients often feel guilty or may be worried that the doctor is going to "yell" at them for not following directions. A good doctor might express some frustration or disappointment, but they should pivot pretty quickly to addressing the patient's concerns.

Should the therapist themselves ever talk to the doctor? Absolutely! There are lots of circumstances in which direct communication between the therapist and the gastroenterologist can be very helpful. As in all other communication about protected health information, be sure to get your patient's consent to release information and help the patient understand *why* you want to talk to their doctor (to educate yourself, to advocate for the patient, etc.) and what the limits of the conversation will be. A few physicians may be surprised or defensive or even resentful of what they see as a boundary crossing, but the vast majority of gastroenterologists I have worked with really appreciate active collaboration. Many times patients have been more honest or clear with me about pain, fatigue, or other symptoms. I've inquired about anemia and iron infusions and had the physician respond with "Sure, that would be great, let me see if the insurance will approve it." I've suggested a fecal calprotectin test when the patient was still symptomatic on a first-line treatment and had the physician say "Oh, that's a good idea!" I've let a doctor know about three episodes of possible SBO in a young patient and had the physician say "I had no idea! Let's get her in here stat for an MRE." I've even suggested the possibility of considering a neuromodulator (especially antidepressants from the SNRI (serotonin norepinephrine reuptake inhibitor) or tricyclic class) and had physicians say "Yeah, I suggested that a few months ago. They didn't want to take it. If you can convince the patient, that would be great." Of course, therapists need to stay within the boundaries of their own competence. But a little bit of knowledge can go a long way when it comes to collaboration and patient advocacy. At the very least, picking up the phone to speak to the doctor to educate yourself about their treatment plan and their understanding of the patient's current status and prognosis can be surprisingly informative and helpful. In fully integrated behavioral health care settings, where therapists with specialized GI knowledge are embedded in gastroenterology departments, this kind of information exchange takes place all the time, both formally and informally. Try to establish at least a modicum of collaboration with the treating physician, even if you are entirely outside the medical system the doctor works in. If you are respectful they will typically appreciate it. One gastroenterologist I spoke to followed a consult with a hopeful "Can I just refer ALL my patients to you?" Sadly, I had to demur. But if there were enough of us out there, then she *could* have referred all of her patients to one of us.

Dietary Interventions

One of the biggest myths about GI disorders is that there is an ideal diet that will reduce or resolve symptoms for most or all people. IBD patients understandably almost always ask their doctors for recommendations about food and diet as a way to control their symptoms and improve or even cure their disease, and you'd think there would be sensible, evidence based advice that doctors could give. Unfortunately, there is much less scientific or medical evidence regarding the impact of diet on IBD than one would hope. In addition, gastroenterologists get remarkably little training about nutrition. Many are becoming more open to recommending and supporting dietary interventions, but some are still dismissive, or just don't know much about it. Medicine is highly siloed, and food is the realm of registered dieticians, some of whom are fabulous and know a lot about IBD, and some of whom aren't and don't. If your patient wants to work with an expert, be sure they find a registered dietician (which is a highly skilled profession, regulated by law, and trained in treating clinical disorders). The term "nutritionist" can mean almost anything and some people have very little training at all. Of course, it can be a challenge to find a good dietician, and many insurance companies won't cover the cost, which is infuriating. But it is still worth the effort.

It would be really nice if there were clear cut, scientifically sound recommendations about how to manage diet to minimize inflammation and IBD symptoms. Unfortunately, we're just not there yet. We do know that a traditional "Western" diet high in processed food, sugar, and saturated fat and low in fiber, whole grains, and vegetables, has terrible effects on the intestinal microbiome and is associated with greater risk for *developing* IBD. We also know that dietary changes can impact the diversity of the microbiome and immune system reactivity, and *may* turn out to be an important adjunctive therapy for people with IBD. Sadly, doing the kind of research necessary to establish the efficacy and the mechanisms of change in specific diets is very difficult. You need a LOT of people who are willing to eat controlled diets and log everything they put into their mouth for a long time. They also need to be willing to give blood and poop samples so the researchers can actually track the impact of the dietary intervention on inflammation and the microbiome. Although we're learning more every day, we still don't really know enough to make specific, targeted recommendations that will work for everyone. That leaves most folks with IBD to turn to nonmedical resources (like the internet) for advice. Unfortunately, most of the patient-targeted dietary recommendations on the internet focus on *restricting* foods or food groups and are highly conflicting and inconsistent. This is particularly concerning because people with IBD often suffer from nutrient malabsorption, so eliminating whole classes of foods often makes malnutrition and nutrient deficiencies *worse*. The biggest concern for people with IBD should be *getting sufficient nutrition*. This means that IBD patients should follow the least restrictive diet possible. If they do end up "cutting" a food or food group, they may need to add in supplements or food substitutes to ensure that they're getting sufficient calories, vitamins, minerals, proteins, fats, and carbohydrates, *all* of which are necessary for life, health, and vitality.

Fiber

One piece of advice that is generally useful for just about all patients with an IBD is to consider adding a soluble fiber supplement to their diet. First, one needs to understand the difference between soluble and insoluble fiber. Fiber is the part of many foods that we cannot fully digest, but it comes in two completely different types. Insoluble fiber does not dissolve in water and passes through the digestive system largely unchanged. It adds "bulk" to stool and is indeed "hard to digest." It is found in the bran of many grains, in the skins and seeds of fruits and vegetables, and in the stalks and leaves of most plant foods. So tomato skins, lettuce leaves, wheat bran, and celery stalks are mostly composed of insoluble fiber. Patients with an IBD will usually want to consume insoluble fiber only in moderation. It increases the volume of stool and decreases transit time (makes food waste move through faster), and tends to make diarrhea and urgency worse. Ironically it can also worsen constipation for IBD patients, since it adds bulk to stool that may already be too hard, dry, and backed up to pass easily. Too much insoluble fiber can also increase the risk of bowel obstructions.

Soluble fiber, on the other hand, dissolves in water, and turns into a gel-like sponge that holds together and gives stool shape while keeping it soft and slippery. As a result, soluble fiber tends to be helpful for both diarrhea and constipation. If your patient is experiencing urgency, and chronic, frequent watery diarrhea, suggest a soluble fiber supplement. It will slow transit time and give stool shape and form, reducing urgency and watery stool. If your patient is struggling with hard, dry stool that is difficult to pass, suggest a soluble fiber supplement. It will soften stool and make it wet and slippery, helping it to pass more easily without straining. Interestingly, soluble fiber is typically fermented by symbiotic bacteria in the gut, making it an important pre-biotic food that helps maintain a healthy microbiome.

Soluble fiber supplements come in a variety of types from a variety of sources. I generally don't recommend psyllium based products (like Metamucil) or inulin (from chicory root) based products because psyllium and inulin are both fairly highly fermentable and can contribute to uncomfortable gas as they are digested by bacteria in the colon. I prefer wheat dextrin products (like Benefiber) that are only moderately fermentable, but still feed friendly symbiotic bacteria like bifidobacteria and lactobacillus. It dissolves completely in water or any semi-liquid food. It has no taste and barely any "mouth feel." Most people won't notice it's there at all and it is typically quite well tolerated. If even those products cause gas, then I recommend Citrucel (methylcellulose) which is the least fermentable supplement. I do not recommend Sunfiber, which is based on guar gum. Guar gum is a common emulsifier used in many foods (such as ice cream) to enhance mouthfeel and texture, and to prevent crystallization. There is increasing evidence that emulsifiers such as carrageenan and guar gum may actually contribute to inflammation in the gut.

Restrictive Diets

Despite the lack of clear, evidence based guidance, most patients with IBD will be advised to try various dietary restrictions, and many will experiment with things on their own. The therapist should certainly review with the patient what their diet is like, and may need to encourage the patient to expand their diet, preferably with the guidance of a good dietician. Understanding some of the basic restrictive diets IBD patients are likely to have heard of, or tried, or may be on can be very helpful.

Lactose. Many IBD patients have tried avoiding lactose (found in dairy). IBD patients are no more likely to be lactose intolerant than anyone else in the population, and the risk of lactose intolerance in IBD patients follows the same ethnic/racial/genetic trends as it does for everyone else. If your patient is convinced they are lactose intolerant, have them try Lactaid products. The actual foods (like Lactaid milk), have little to no lactose in them. The tablets (which can be taken immediately before consuming dairy products) contain the enzyme lactase, which breaks down the lactose in the food before it causes problems. Yogurt and hard cheeses contain relatively little lactose (because it has already been broken down by bacterial cultures). They are generally perfectly fine to eat. There is little reason to encourage patients to get the lactose tolerance hydrogen breath test done. These tests don't correlate all that well with actual intolerance, and many people who tolerate lactose just fine will still "fail" the test. Nevertheless, there is evidence from crossover placebo trials that lactase supplements will significantly reduce exhaled hydrogen in response to lactose consumption. There is certainly no harm in encouraging patients to use Lactaid products if they believe that lactose makes their symptoms worse.

Gluten. Many IBD patients have also tried avoiding gluten (a protein found in wheat, rye, and barley). With respect to gluten, IBD patients *are* at increased risk for celiac disease (or true gluten intolerance) which is another autoimmune disorder. If they do test positive for celiac disease, they absolutely must avoid all sources of gluten. Untreated celiac disease can result in irreversible damage to the villi of the small intestine. On the other hand, if they do *not* have celiac disease, gluten is highly unlikely to exacerbate inflammation. Many people have come to believe that lots of humans can't "tolerate" gluten (known as non-celiac gluten sensitivity or NCGS) but the actual evidence for this is inconsistent at best. About a third of patients with Crohn's believe that they have NCGS, but again there is no confirmatory test for this, and patients often seize on popular restrictive diets that they hope will provide them with relief. There are no well-done prospective randomized controlled trials of a gluten-free diet in IBD. Many IBD diets (see below) encourage avoiding wheat, but generally because of the specific carbohydrates wheat contains, *not* because of the gluten. I typically encourage my patients to stop avoiding gluten, unless, of course, they actually have celiac disease.

Low FODMAP Diet. The Low FODMAP Diet is a *highly* restrictive diet. There is some evidence that it is helpful (in the short term) for secondary IBS in patients with IBD in remission who are still experiencing GI symptoms. There is much less evidence that it is helpful for IBD patients more generally. FODMAP stands for "Fermentable **O**ligo-, **D**i- and **M**ono-saccharides and **P**olyols." These are all carbohydrates that are broken down, or *fermented* by the intestinal microbiome—those symbiotic bacteria that live in the gut. In fact, these are *all* the *prebiotic* foods that nourish our microbiome. High FODMAP foods *do* reliably cause more gas and water content in the gut as a by-product of the fermentation process. Eliminating or severely restricting those foods can reduce the volume of stool by reducing the gas and water in the gut, and may help control diarrhea. It's worth noting that they don't cause any more gas and water for people with IBS or IBD than they do for anyone else. It's just that people with chronic GI issues are much more bothered by the gas and water.

The diet attempts to eliminate all the carbohydrates which are fermented during digestion and may exacerbate gas, flatulence, cramping, and diarrhea. It is *extremely* restrictive and difficult to follow, and it's difficult to get good nutrition on it. Patients really must work with a knowledgeable dietician if they want to try it. In the strict elimination phase (which lasts six to eight weeks) patients must avoid all dairy (lactose), wheat and rye (because of the fructans they contain, *not* gluten, which is a protein), all legumes (all beans, including soy, peas, chickpeas and lentils), most sweeteners, and many fruits and vegetables (including onions and garlic, apples, pears, melons, stone fruits (including peaches and cherries), broccoli, cauliflower, and many others including avocado, mushrooms, and beets). The FODMAP Diet does allow *some* fruits (like bananas, citrus, and blueberries) and vegetables (including carrots, eggplant, corn, celery, spinach, and lettuce). But overall, it tends to be fairly meat heavy and fairly low fiber, which is ironic given all the evidence about the importance of eating a low meat, high fiber diet. It's really hard to stick to if you're a vegetarian, because it eliminates all the legumes and dairy, so it's very hard to consume enough complete protein (you can still eat eggs).

There is mounting evidence that following a low FODMAP diet can reduce discomfort and improve quality of life in IBD patients, especially if they have secondary IBS and the IBD is in remission. One short term study that lasted six weeks suggested that strict adherence to the Low FODMAP Diet could improve both patient reported symptoms and objective inflammatory markers in the stool. BUT! There are some important caveats. First, the effect of restricting high FODMAP foods on the microbiome is worrisome. Whole species of "good" bacteria die out because they starve to death. Second, it's such a restrictive diet that it's really quite hard to follow, and it's hard to get adequate nutrition on it under the best of circumstances. Even Peter Gibson, one of the originators of the diet, warns that "The risk of compromising nutritional status with a restrictive diet must be seriously considered especially as undernutrition is already common in this patient population. ... As undernutrition is common in IBD, the use of restrictive diets should be supervised by a dietitian." [Gibson, P.R. (2017). Use of the low-FODMAP diet in inflammatory bowel disease. *Journal of Gastroenterology and Hepatology.*]]

It's also important to note that patients shouldn't stick to the strict elimination phase of the diet for more than six weeks, for all the reasons listed above. They're supposed to start slowly reintroducing FODMAP containing foods over time until they get back to a reasonably varied diet.

Specific Carbohydrate Diet. SCD is another highly restrictive diet that eliminates pretty much ALL grains (including wheat, rye, and barley, but ALSO rice, oats, and corn, which are allowed in the Low FODMAP Diet) and starchy tubers (potatoes, sweet potatoes), some legumes, canola oil, all sweeteners, and most dairy products. It does allow most of the vegetables that the Low FODMAP Diet restricts, but it is still very difficult to follow. Most of the evidence supporting it is anecdotal, with a few survey studies thrown in. Nevertheless, some patients are absolutely convinced that following the diet is an important part of their recovery. People who stick to it long term may experience nutrient deficiencies, and should be monitored for vitamin D and calcium, and possible weight loss.

IBD Anti-Inflammatory Diet. IBD-AID is yet another variation on a restrictive diet. This one also restricts specific carbohydrates, including lactose from fresh milk and cheeses, all grains (except oats), and refined sugar, as well as trans-fats (found in partially or fully hydrogenated oil). On the other hand the diet *allows* and even encourages consumption of many other prebiotic and probiotic foods, including yogurt and kefir, aged cheeses, onions and garlic, all vegetables (steamed and pureed if necessary, or baby or micro versions to reduce insoluble fiber load), and legumes. Like the Low FODMAP Diet it is intended to be followed in stages, with the most restrictive phase first, followed by systematic reintroduction, with the maintenance phase being the least restrictive diet possible.

Low Residue Diets. Low residue diets restrict the amount of fiber the patient eats in order to reduce the overall volume of stool. The idea is that low residue foods put less "stress" on the intestines and will pass through the digestive tract more slowly. It is essentially a very low fiber diet, and eliminates most sources of insoluble fiber (the type that doesn't dissolve in water). Insoluble fiber is found in the bran of grains, and in the skins and seeds of fruits and vegetables, as well as in stalks and leaves. Ironically, the low residue diet relies on many of the exact foods that other restrictive diets eliminate, including white bread, pasta, rice, and highly refined cereals (like corn flakes and puffed rice), well cooked potatoes and sweet potatoes, melon, peaches and plums, and dairy products (which are naturally fiber free). Patients still need to avoid beans and legumes, whole grains, many raw vegetables and fruits, fruit and vegetable skins, and nuts and seeds. Doctors will often recommend a low residue diet while a patient is in flare, if a patient has significant strictures or after surgery. But it's not really a good long term solution for most people.

Liquid Diet. There is some evidence that switching to a fully liquid diet, at least for periods of time, can dramatically reduce inflammation and symptoms for pediatric IBD patients. However, there is only modest evidence supporting the use of a total liquid diet or liquid diet supplementation in adults. Nevertheless, some adult patients with both Crohn's and UC find that supplementing occasionally or regularly with a liquid meal replacement eases their symptoms and reduces the burden of frequent diarrhea and urgency. Traditional products like Ensure and Boost are options, but there are a number of other products available as well, including Kate Farms products (which are plant based and organic) and others. In some cases, insurance will actually cover the cost of these meal replacements for patients with IBD.

Enteral Feeding. Some pediatric and young adult IBD patients turn to using liquid diets which can be delivered directly to the stomach via a feeding tube inserted through the nose (called a naso-gastric or NG tube). Kids are remarkably adaptive around this, and the feeding often takes place at night, while they are asleep. While this may make sleepovers impossible, for some kids it is enough to induce remission, and in Europe is used as a first-line treatment for pediatric IBD. It is more problematic for young adults, especially if they need to leave the feeding tube in place rather than removing and reinserting it every day. One young adult I worked with was so ill and underweight during her freshman year of college she wore a naso-gastric tube 24 hours a day. Needless to say, many of her classmates assumed she had a severe eating disorder and she endured a good deal of social exclusion and shame as a result. It is important for the therapist to be alert to the possibility that an adult patient may have a history of using enteral feeding that can be emotionally very complicated, even if it was lifesaving at the time.

In sum, the dietary advice out there for IBD patients is confusing, conflicting, and mostly not well supported by science. This can leave patients feeling demoralized and helpless, or stuck on a highly restrictive diet they are afraid, or even *terrified* of deviating from. I had one patient who was eating nothing but peanut butter and jelly sandwiches on white bread when I started working with her. Not surprisingly, she was anemic, B12 deficient, exhausted, and terribly constipated. It took several months, but she eventually got back to a much more varied and healthful diet which, along with several iron infusions, dramatically improved her energy and mood. If your patient hasn't already done so, you should encourage them to seek the guidance of a registered dietician who is knowledgeable about IBD. Dealing with fear of food, trauma around past feeding or eating issues, social exclusion because they eat a "weird" diet, embarrassment and so on are often core issues for IBD patients, and the therapist needs to be knowledgeable about them.

Steroids

Love 'em or hate 'em, steroids are going to be part of medical management at some point for most patients with an IBD. The two main steroids that would be likely to be prescribed to someone with an IBD are prednisone and budesonide (Entocort or Uceris). Both have significant anti-inflammatory effects while the patient is taking them. They can calm down symptomatic flares and improve GI symptoms significantly, typically inducing remission in a relatively short period of time. This is the "love 'em" part of steroids. Unfortunately, steroids only work while the patient is taking them, and they have a *lot* of side effects, so they should generally only be used in the lowest effective dose for the shortest amount of time possible. Prednisone can be helpful for both Crohn's and UC whereas budesonide (Entocort) is typically used in Crohn's because it is effective at the end of the small intestine (ileum) and the beginning of the colon (cecum). There is a new form of budesonide (Uceris) that can also be used in UC.

It's important for patients to remember that nearly every drug in existence, including aspirin, carries an enormous laundry list of potential side effects, ranging from mildly annoying to downright terrifying. Unfortunately, there is usually no way for a doctor to predict exactly which side effects, if any, will occur, and how severe they will be. Different people may react in completely different ways to the same drug. The only way to know how a specific patient will react is if *they* take the drug. The important thing is to evaluate the risk/benefit profile of any given treatment option objectively, without catastrophizing all the possibilities.

About half of people taking steroids will experience a particular side effect called "moon face" in which the face swells up (due to fatty deposits in the cheeks and temples) and looks much rounder than normal. Doctors consider this a "minor" side effect because it's not dangerous and it usually resolves within a few weeks to a month when the patient stops taking the drug. But most patients *hate* it. It's embarrassing. They don't look like themselves. People might ask them about it. Lots of people say it makes them feel "fat" even when their overall weight hasn't changed. So while doctors might not worry about it because it's just "cosmetic" (not dangerous), patients are often quite distressed by it. My advice to the patient is two-fold. First, remember that it is temporary. Second, if people ask them about it, they should just tell them the truth!

More serious side effects of steroids can include nervousness or agitation, insomnia, slightly worsening depression or in some cases hypomanic mood and behavior, mood swings, psychosis (in vulnerable individuals), greater vulnerability to infections, and long term osteoporosis or weakened bones. This is the real "hate 'em" side of steroids, and it's why patients should be on them at the lowest dose possible for the shortest time possible. That said, steroids can dramatically improve health related quality of life, and can give the gut a chance to calm down and heal, which can give other medications a chance to take effect. As with any choice, patients have to weigh the potential risks and benefits of both taking the steroid, AND the potential risks and benefits of NOT taking the steroid. One of the advantages of budesonide (over prednisone) is that it tends to have fewer systemic (whole body) effects, and concentrates the effects in the intestines where it's needed, so doctors will typically opt for that if they think it will be effective, reserving prednisone for more severe flares. Indeed, Uceris (budesonide for UC) also comes in a suppository or foam that can be inserted directly into the rectum, confining its effects right where it is needed.

I like to remind my patients that if their doctor recommends short term use of steroids, they should go for it. Some people get so worried about long term consequences (like osteoporosis) that they would rather endure severe pain, weight loss, fatigue, and other symptoms rather than take steroids. I remind people that this is faulty logic. If your gut is badly inflamed, you're at high risk for nutritional deficiencies, which in itself puts you at higher risk for osteoporosis! I strongly encourage people to take steroids recommended by their doctor for a time to get their IBD under better control in the short term. It can dramatically improve quality of life while they work with their doctor to come up with a good long term solution that will help keep them in remission when they wean off the steroid.

Some patients with IBD have the opposite problem—they grow to rely on steroids to keep their IBD under control and are very reluctant to wean off them. They are convinced that the steroid "works" (which of course it does) and may be very reluctant to get off the steroid in favor of a more effective and ultimately safer longer-term treatment. Some GI docs have a hard time not prescribing steroids in the face of patient distress and symptoms. Others report being frustrated with patients who "demand" steroids and refuse to consider other medication options. In either of these cases, it can be important to consult with the gastroenterologist and to work collaboratively with them and the patient toward getting them onto a more appropriate medication regimen.

Other Medications

The list of other medications that can be used to treat IBD is long and ever changing, and even a comprehensive review would probably be out of date pretty quickly. Nevertheless, there are a few standards that are worth touching on, with the understanding that this list will by necessity be incomplete.

Along with steroids, the first-line treatment for UC in the colon (but not Crohn's disease) is typically an anti-inflammatory medication called

mesalamine (5-aminosalicylic acid or 5-ASA). Mesalamine can be taken as a pill, or given as an enema or suppository (the most common route in ulcerative proctitis, since it works directly in the rectum). You can remain on mesalamine for years, and many people with mild UC find that this is sufficient treatment for them. Patients will need to have basic labs done periodically to check on kidney function, but in general mesalamine is quite safe. One advantage of it is that it has relatively few systemic side effects, and mostly exerts its effects directly in the colon.

If patients do not have a sufficient response to mesalamine (or if they have Crohn's disease) then they will typically need infusion or injection therapy, in the class of "biologic" medications. Biologics work by blocking chemical messages from the immune system that trigger a cascade of inflammation in patients with IBD. These include some of the most common medications IBD patients might take. The most well known are **Humira** (adalimumab), **Remicade/Inflectra/Renflexis** (infliximab), **Entyvio** (vedolizumab), and **Stelara** (ustekinumab), but others include **Enbrel** (etanercept), **Cimzia** (certolizumab pegol), **Simponi** (golimumab), and **Skyrizi** (risankizumab). Because Humira is one of the oldest, and is off patent, insurance companies will often insist that a patient *fail* a trial of Humira before being allowed to try one of the newer medications. *All* the biologic therapies suppress the immune system to some degree. The most common side effects include infections (which can be serious), headaches, rashes, upper respiratory infections, sinusitis, cough, and sore throat. TNF blockers (which include Humira, Remicade, Enbrel, Cimzia, and Simponi) and IL/IL blockers (including Stelara) also increase the risk of lymphomas and non-melanoma skin cancers. Remicade and Entyvio must be given by infusion at an infusion center, but the others can be administered by injection that patients can learn to give themselves.

Entyvio prevents white blood cells that cause inflammation from entering the intestines. It can only be given by infusion. Stelara targets several proteins associated with inflammation in the gut. It needs to be given by infusion initially, but then the patient can self-inject it after the initial onboarding doses. Both Stelara and Entyvio can be quite effective at promoting mucosal healing in both UC and Crohn's, even in people who have failed to respond to earlier treatment with anti-TNFs. Patients will typically need treatment every six to eight weeks, but once a regular dosing schedule is established, most people tolerate these drugs quite well, and they often get people into remission and keep them there.

Xeljanz (tofacitinib) and **Zeposia** (ozanimod) are anti-inflammatory pills (the only "advanced" therapies that are like biologics as of this writing that can be taken orally) that can be used to treat moderate to severe UC.

Another form of medication are the "immunomodulators" (**Imuran** (azathioprine); methotrexate, thiopurines, or **Purixan** (mercaptopurine or 6-MP)). These are rarely used on their own, but might be given in combination with other medications.

Even more important than a basic primer on the medications themselves, however, is a good understanding of the general emotional and practical issues that might come up for people.

Mode of Delivery. Most IBD drugs (the anti-TNFs and all the biologics except Xeljanz and Zeposia) must be taken as an injection or an infusion. This can mean going to a center to get the infusions, or learning to give oneself injections at home. Infusion centers can be inconvenient to get to and it can be quite time consuming to get it done. (It typically takes at least two hours for the infusion itself, not counting transportation, or the time to set up and check out.) The patient's main GI doctor will need to be affiliated with a particular infusion center, which may or may not be part of a specific hospital system. Some insurance companies will approve home infusion, but it depends on the patient's individual plan. While injectable drugs can be significantly more convenient, they have their own complications. For folks who don't have a background in medicine, learning to give themselves shots can be intimidating, although most people get the hang of it pretty quickly and it starts to seem routine. Other issues include pain or discomfort during the injection. Newer formulations of some drugs (like citrate-free Humira) have dramatically reduced the burning pain many people used to associate with the injection. This has been a huge boon to IBD patients everywhere.

Actual Delivery. Injectable drugs typically need to be delivered by post from mail order pharmacies. Some need to be kept cold (like Stelara) and if you work outside the home it may be tricky to figure out when to have it delivered so that you can get it into the fridge as soon as possible. Fortunately, new evidence suggests that this (very expensive) drug won't be spoiled even if the cold chain is briefly interrupted. It keeps for 30 days. So patients should try not to fret too much if it ends up sitting on their front porch for a few hours until they get home. They also don't need to worry about the exact temperature in their fridge.

Potential Side Effects. Many of the powerful drugs used to treat IBD have potential side effects that can be scary or even life threatening. Many patients are reluctant to even try a medication because of the possibility (however slight) of liver or kidney toxicity, infection, or cancer. Those concerns are real, and a therapist can certainly empathize with the devil's choice patients must make when it comes to managing their disease. Patients should discuss with their doctor what steps can be taken to minimize the chances of experiencing these adverse effects. For example, doctors will typically want to monitor kidney and/or liver health with regular blood work, and may decide to adjust the dose, or switch to a new medicine entirely if there are issues. As always, patients need to consider not just the risks of taking the drug, but also the risks of NOT taking the drug. Several IBD drugs increase the risk of non-melanoma skin cancer (NMSC) in particular. You can minimize this risk by wearing sunscreen and visiting your dermatologist yearly to get checked. If caught early, NMSC is typically easy to remove and the five year survival rate is 100%. Remember that untreated IBD itself can increase the risk of colon cancer significantly. So the patient needs to take their total cancer risk into account in making their decisions. If their quality of life is really taking a beating because their IBD isn't under good control, then not pursuing medical options out of fear of *potential* side effects is probably unwise.

Women who are considering pregnancy often have major concerns about continuing to take their IBD medication. Many women prefer to stop IBD therapy before or when they get pregnant for fear of side effects. However, this actually places the mother and fetus at *higher* risk for complications. IBD flares and having active inflammation in the body isn't good for Mom or developing baby. Many studies have now shown that it is actually much safer for both Mom and baby if Mom stays on her IBD medication (with the notable exceptions of Xeljanz and Zeposia). You can also safely nurse on these medications (again, except for Xeljanz and Zeposia).

Remember that most people are much more upset about the thought of *doing* something that ends up having a bad result than they are about *not doing* something that ends up having a bad result. Technically called *commission error bias*, we don't like *committing acts* that we end up regretting. Weirdly, errors of omission (failing to act) don't usually stir up quite the same feelings of guilt and regret. It's odd, because failing to act can have consequences that are just as bad. So people tend to worry a lot more about deciding to *take* Remicade or Stelara and then regretting it because they developed an adverse effect, than they worry about deciding *not* to manage their IBD aggressively, and having bad outcomes as a result. Even though this bias toward judging sins of commission more harshly is pretty universal, it's actually pretty illogical. They are both choices to behave in a certain way that end up having consequences.

Lots of folks with an IBD are tough—they can tolerate a lot of discomfort, fatigue, skin lesions, joint pain, diarrhea: you name it. I have tremendous respect for people who manage to go about their lives (even if in a somewhat limited way) carrying the burdens of an active IBD. But I strongly encourage my patients to consider their overall quality of life when making decisions about medication management. If medication can drastically improve their quality of life, it's almost certainly worth giving it a try.

It's also worth remembering that new medications are being developed and tested for inflammatory bowel diseases every day. Sometimes new medicines become available in limited ways to people in clinical trials or through special restricted distribution programs. Sometimes it isn't clear whether the benefits of a medication will outweigh the risks associated with using it. Obviously, a patient's doctor should stay abreast of all the latest developments in medicines for IBD. The doctor should also help patients think through clearly the potential costs and benefits of any particular medication regimen, given the type and severity of their IBD, the location of the inflammation, the impact of the IBD on their quality of life and overall health and so on. We can all fervently hope that new drug discoveries are on the horizon that will bring a true cure. This isn't just wishful thinking. After all, ten years ago hepatitis C was considered hard to treat and almost impossible to cure—and the medication regimens that existed had terrible side effects for lots of people who tried them (including suicidal depression—yikes!). Today there are several medications that can cure up to 98% of patients with hepatitis C and have *very* benign side effect profiles. It's really amazing when you think about it. So patients should keep asking their doctor about new trials and new developments. Maybe one day soon we'll be able to cure IBD too, without the risk of serious side effects.

Surgical Treatment

The sad truth is that even with good medical management, up to 25% of UC patients and up to 50% of Crohn's patients will require corrective or even lifesaving surgery at some point in their lives. Worrying about the possibility of needing surgery, deciding whether to undergo surgery or not, and making decisions about the type of surgery they undergo is often an underlying stressor for IBD patients, and something that is often worth exploring in therapy. This section provides a basic primer on the types of surgical interventions that IBD patients might undergo and some of the risks and potential benefits you can help them think through.

Endoscopic Balloon Dilation and Strictureplasty. Recall that IBD patients are vulnerable to the development of strictures—narrow spots in the intestines caused by scar tissue that is thickened and rigid. Because strictures put people at risk of developing bowel obstructions, and can generally cause slowed motility, difficulty digesting fiberous foods, and cramping discomfort, doctors will sometimes suggest attempting to widen the stricture. One procedure is endoscopic balloon dilation. It is minimally invasive, fairly safe, and conserves the bowel tissues. It is used for very short strictures, and does not require any incision, as it is carried out with an endoscope that is inserted through the anus. Unfortunately, it doesn't always work, and many patients will ultimately require corrective surgery within three to four years. However, it can certainly buy time and make people more comfortable.

Another procedure is called strictureplasty. This is, in theory, the least invasive type of surgical procedure done for IBD patients, and involves making an incision in the abdomen and then either stretching the stricture mechanically, or making incisions in the wall of the intestine to widen or bypass the stricture. Ideally, no intestine is removed.

Resection. When portions of the intestines are so inflamed, ulcerated, or damaged that they cannot heal even with aggressive medical management, surgeons may strongly suggest resecting, or removing the damaged length of the bowel. Ideally, they will be able to sew the two ends of healthy tissue together, and the person will heal and be able to eat and defecate normally. Depending on how much tissue is removed, a simple resection may help the person feel *much* better after they recover. Often they are in significantly less pain and may be at lower risk of an obstruction. However, even a highly successful resection will have consequences. The join where the two ends were sewn together is called an *anastomosis* and is often the site of new scarring, narrowing, or inflammation. It can also be difficult subsequently to get scopes through the anastomosis, depending on exactly where it is and how it is positioned relative to the normal twists and turns of the gut. Depending on the portion of the gut that is removed, you can end up with specific nutritional deficiencies or bile acid diarrhea. (This is especially likely if they have to remove part or all of the ileum, which is the last section of the small intestine. That's where both vitamin B12 and excess bile acid are absorbed.) If the patient has had an *ileal resection* and is still experiencing watery diarrhea, ask them if they have talked to their physician about taking a *bile acid sequestrant* (brand names include Colestipol, Welchol, and Questran). This is a medication that binds to excess bile acid and keeps it from making it into the colon, where it can cause a build-up of water and electrolytes in the stool. Bile acid sequestrants come in a gritty, resinous powder that can be mixed with yogurt or applesauce, or in pill form. The pills are fairly large and can be hard to swallow, so be sure to encourage the patient to get the brand name (which has rounded edges and a slippery coating), not the generic. You have to time them carefully around any other medications, which can be inconvenient, but if bile acid is a problem, these drugs can help significantly with diarrhea.

Most patients are very anxious about undergoing a resection, and may not be convinced that they need it, or that the risks are worth it. Some patients are very glad they did it, and feel *much* better afterwards. Some even wonder why they waited so long and wish they had done it earlier. However, like any surgery, it comes with real risks. Depending on how much of the small intestine needs to be removed, patients run the risk of developing *short bowel syndrome.* Ironically, the main symptoms of short bowel syndrome are diarrhea, cramping, fatigue, and malnutrition secondary to poor absorption— many of the very symptoms caused by Crohn's disease itself. People with moderate to severe short bowel will often need nutritional support, supplementation, and a somewhat restrictive diet. Sometimes during surgery the surgeon finds that there simply isn't enough healthy bowel tissue to reconnect. This can lead to a much more extreme or invasive procedure than what the patient was expecting and is a feared outcome for many patients with IBD who elect to undergo surgery.

J-pouch. The most common corrective surgery recommended for patients with UC is a proctocolectomy with ileal pouch–anal anastomosis, or j-pouch surgery. In the procedure, the surgeon removes the entire colon and the rectum, and then reconnects the end of the small intestine (the ileum) to form an internal pouch (shaped like a J) and connects it to the anus. The anal sphincter muscle is left intact. Most individuals will have to have a temporary ileostomy while the new j-pouch heals. A hole, or stoma, is created in the front of the abdomen and a loop of small intestine will be opened up to it, allowing waste to come out and be collected in an ostomy bag that is attached to the abdomen using adhesive. Once the j-pouch has healed (typically eight to twelve weeks later), the ostomy will be reversed and the stoma will be closed. Living with an ostomy, even temporarily, is something many IBD patients dread. Recovery from the j-pouch procedure can take some time, and the muscles in the resulting pouch need to learn to store stool and then squeeze it out. (Remember, the ileum normally absorbs lots of nutrients and then passes food waste along into the colon. It's not really designed to simply hold on to stool.) However, the main advantage of this procedure is that once the patient has recovered, they may be permanently cured of UC. UC only occurs in the colon, so once the colon is gone, so is the inflammation. Moreover, the patient should be able to eat and defecate normally, although they may always have to alter their diet somewhat in favor of lower fiber foods.

Unfortunately, up to 80% of patients with a j-pouch will develop a complication called *pouchitis* at least once, with anywhere from 25% to 50% having recurring or chronic pouchitis. Pouchitis is inflammation or infection in the new pouch/rectum. Signs and symptoms of pouchitis can include diarrhea, abdominal pain, joint pain, cramps, and fever. Other signs and symptoms include an increased number of bowel movements, urgency, nighttime stool leakage, and difficulty controlling bowel movements (up to and including fecal incontinence). It is typically treated with antibiotics, leading to resolution of the problem, but in many cases it becomes chronic. Thus, about half of patients with this surgery will go on to lead healthy lives with relatively normal digestion and elimination. Indeed, historical data suggest that around 90% of patients will maintain a "functional" pouch after 30 years. But anywhere from a quarter to a half of patients will not have great outcomes. This is incredibly frustrating and demoralizing for patients. Some things can be done prophylactically to prevent the likelihood of pouchitis, including probiotic supplementation after surgery for up to a year. This appears to reduce dysbiosis that can contribute to pouchitis. But some patients will require other treatments, including the usual round of steroids and even biologic medications from the TNF blocker class—meaning patients are sometimes right back where they started. A few will ultimately elect to abandon normal defecation and opt for a permanent ostomy instead.

Permanent Ostomy. This is the worst case scenario for many IBD patients, and it is the treatment of last resort for patients with severe symptoms that cannot be managed with medication and more conservative surgeries. In this case, so much of the bowel tissue is damaged that segmental resection or j-pouch procedures are impossible. The only option is to remove a significant length of the bowel and create a permanent ostomy.

Adjusting to an ostomy is complicated. There is some evidence that for many people quality of life ultimately improves because they are no longer sick and in pain all the time. But there is no question that learning to live with a bag of poop on the outside of your tummy just under your clothes takes *a lot* of emotional and practical work. If you have a patient who has recently had an ostomy and is still struggling with it, strongly encourage them to find a local support group, and to consult with ostomy experts (typically GI nurses or occupational therapists) who are knowledgeable about different pouching systems and the care of the stoma (the flesh around the new hole in the abdominal wall). On the practical side, patients worry a good deal about the bag leaking. Some find that they are allergic to the adhesive in some bag systems but not others. Some prefer to have bags that can be emptied while still attached (to minimize changing the adhesive "wafer" which can irritate the skin) while others strongly prefer to use closed bag systems that can be removed and thrown away. Talking to experienced ostomates can go a long way toward helping patients make the adjustment successfully.

Women in particular (but men also) worry about the bag being visible under their clothes, or emitting odors (or worse). Many appearance/body issues can trigger social anxiety, self-consciousness, and body image problems. But poop really is singularly taboo and icky for people to talk about. Validate that for your patient, but work with them to find ways to explain it and give people the head's up when necessary. Intimacy in particular can feel very challenging. If the patient has the procedure done while they're still single, it can make dating incredibly daunting and embarrassing. When do you tell a potential partner? Over dinner on the first date? On the second or third date when you consider more than a quick good night cheek peck? When the clothes actually start to come off? Telling a new partner about an ostomy can be scary, but it shouldn't get in the way of a patient's dating life. Although rejection is always a possibility, I suggest that they find a way to raise the issue *before* they end up in the bedroom with someone. Indeed, one way to positively frame an ostomy is that it is a great *test* of any new partner. If they are considerate, understanding, and sensitive about it, that speaks well of their character and their potential as a partner. If they are rude, insensitive, or rejecting, then the patient wouldn't want to partner with them anyway. Even in happily partnered people, sexuality can take a real hit when one person has a new ostomy. Fortunately, there are many wonderful resources (like www.ostomysecrets.com) that sell fun, functional (and even sexy) underwear and swimwear designed specifically for ostomates.

Common Concerns

Leakage

Shit happens, literally. Unfortunately, leakages do happen, although they are almost always preventable. The majority of ostomates blame leakages on personal mistakes such as not checking to make sure the clip or seal on their pouch is tight enough, using a new pouching system to which they haven't adjusted, or having a pouch system that is not compatible with their particular stoma shape and/or size.

The main solution is to be proactive. Encourage your patient to be careful and methodical when applying and sealing a new pouch. If they're ordering a new pouch system, do a "trial run" while they finish out the supply of their old system: they can wear the new system at times they're not planning to leave the house and see how they adjust.

Many ostomates report issues with night leakages. To avoid this, they can use appliances with larger bags/pouches for nighttime hours and, if using an open-end system, drain before bed.

Like fecal incontinence, people are often terrified of leakage. The key to surviving without being overwhelmed by worry is to help your patient remember that even if their pouch does leak, it is *not* a catastrophe. Inconvenient? Absolutely. A bit embarrassing? Certainly. But they know how to clean up. If they are experimenting with a new system, they should keep a change of clothes in their car or stash it at work.

Blockages

Sometimes, stool can accumulate and plug up the stoma, causing a blockage. This is more likely to occur in people with ileostomies, although colostomy patients can have blockages too. When a patient has a blockage, their stoma will be inactive or output will be unusually watery. To try and loosen up the stool, they can try taking a warm bath to relax their abdominal muscles, getting on the floor in a knee to chest position, or massaging the area around the stoma. If the stoma is inactive for four to six hours, accompanied by cramping or nausea, they should call their doctor. To avoid blockages, they may need to make sure to chew their food well, especially when eating high residue foods such as pineapple, nuts, coconut, celery, and corn.

Catastrophic Thoughts

Catastrophic thoughts can occur about lots of different things in lots of different situations for everyone, IBD or not. Catastrophic thoughts about ostomies may seem particularly scary and plausible. But a little consideration of the evidence may put many fears to rest. For example, patients may think that *everyone* notices their ostomy bag under their clothing. But do they really? Let's look at the evidence. According to the UOAA (United Ostomy Associations of America), 1.5–2 million people have ostomies. That's a lot of folks out there! Early on in my career I had a client with an ostomy and I had *no idea* until his wife told me. (They were actually in treatment to help her manage her obsessive-compulsive disorder, and its impact on the family, and not specifically for him.) So, chances are you've come across at least one ostomate and *never noticed*.

Patients also may think that everyone hears that gurgle from their stoma or the release of gas. Remind your patient that even people without ostomies or IBD make the occasional stomach grumble or gas burble. Most likely if someone even notices the noises or gas, they'll attribute it to an everyday phenomenon or to someone else.

Patients may well think that their ostomy is ugly or disgusting in some way. They might be surprised by how invisible it is to others, even if they're looking right at it. Patients might even be surprised by the degree to which people who love them see their ostomy as *part* of the person they love. In the eyes of love, even stomas can look like dimples.

The more we can destigmatize IBD and the various treatment options they entail, the better it will be for everyone. I like to remind patients that before the 1970s the Federal Communications Commission (FCC) didn't let people say the word *cancer* on TV. It was considered too stigmatized and disturbing to even talk about. In fact, the first time a character on a TV show even had a cancer scare was in 1973 on *All in the Family*. And even the folks at that groundbreaking show (created by Norman Lear and starring Jean Stapleton as Edith) were concerned about it and debated a *lot* about whether to run the story line. That seems ridiculous and unimaginable now. We can all look forward to the day when IBD are no longer stigmatized as much as well.

Summary

IBD are treated with a range of interventions, from various restrictive diets, through a wide variety of medications, and up to surgical interventions that may be relatively minimal or truly invasive and life altering. As in any field of medicine, every potential treatment has both potential benefits and potential risks. In the case of IBD, many of the medications (steroids, immunosuppressants) have very real possible adverse effects including increased risk of infection, osteoporosis, liver or kidney toxicity, and even cancer. Patients will often appreciate help from a knowledgeable therapist to sort through their options and think through the balance of possible risks and benefits of various treatments. With respect to food, it is important to remember that none of the restrictive diets have particularly good support for their efficacy from well done clinical trials, but some may indeed provide symptomatic relief. Therapists can help patients understand the possible mechanisms of action and the potential benefits (and risks!) of restrictive diets and of fiber supplementation.

Therapists can also advocate for patients, and can facilitate good communication between the patient and the doctor. Patients are often far more willing to discuss a variety of things related to their IBD management—their symptoms, any side effects they are experiencing, their fears, and their reluctance to try something new—with their therapist than they are with their doctor. Therapists can provide a very useful bridge between the doctor and the patient, and can often translate back and forth between the lay language of the patient and the technical jargon of the doctor. Therapists often have considerably more time to talk about these things (up to an hour a week!) than physicians do (who may only 15 minutes with the patient every three months). As always, the therapist should be mindful of the boundaries of their own competence, and should always defer to the doctor's knowledge and expertise. But being willing to have these conversations (with both patients and doctors) in an informed way can be enormously useful and can facilitate effective, collaborative care.

Bibliography

Abdalla, M. I., Sandler, R. S., Kappelman, M. D., Martin, C. F., Chen, W., Anton, K. & Long, M. D. (2016). The impact of ostomy on quality of life and functional status of Crohn's disease patients. *Inflammatory Bowel Diseases, 22*(11), 2658–2664.

Akiyama, S., Rai, V. & Rubin, D. T. (2021). Pouchitis in inflammatory bowel disease: a review of diagnosis, prognosis, and treatment. *Intestinal Research, 19*(1), 1–11.

Alenezi, A., McGrath, I., Kimpton, A. & Livesay, K. (2021). Quality of life among ostomy patients: A narrative literature review. *Journal of Clinical Nursing, 30*(21–22), 3111–3123.

Beaugerie, L., Rahier, J. F. & Kirchgesner, J. (2020). Predicting, preventing, and managing treatment-related complications in patients with inflammatory bowel diseases. *Clinical Gastroenterology and Hepatology, 18*(6), 1324–1335.

Bettenworth, D., Gustavsson, A., Atreja, A., Lopez, R., Tysk, C., Van Assche, G. & Rieder, F. (2017). A pooled analysis of efficacy, safety, and long-term outcome of endoscopic balloon dilation therapy for patients with stricturing Crohn's disease. *Inflammatory Bowel Diseases, 23*(1), 133–142.

Chiba, M., Nakane, K. & Komatsu, M. (2019). Westernized diet is the most ubiquitous environmental factor in inflammatory bowel disease. *The Permanente Journal, 23.*

Dalal, R. L., Shen, B. & Schwartz, D. A. (2018). Management of pouchitis and other common complications of the pouch. *Inflammatory Bowel Diseases, 24*(5), 989–996.

Dietz, D. W., Laureti, S., Strong, S. A., Hull, T. L., Church, J., Remzi, F. H., ... & Fazio, V. W. (2001). Safety and longterm efficacy of strictureplasty in 314 patients with obstructing small bowel Crohn's disease. *Journal of the American College of Surgeons, 192*(3), 330–337.

Gallo, G., Kotze, P. G. & Spinelli, A. (2018). Surgery in ulcerative colitis: When? How? *Best Practice & Research Clinical Gastroenterology, 32,* 71–78.

Gibson, P. R. (2017). Use of the low-FODMAP diet in inflammatory bowel disease. *Journal of Gastroenterology and Hepatology, 32,* 40–42.

Knight-Sepulveda, K., Kais, S., Santaolalla, R. & Abreu, M. T. (2015). Diet and inflammatory bowel disease. *Gastroenterology & Hepatology, 11*(8), 511.

Lewis, J. D. & Abreu, M. T. (2017). Diet as a trigger or therapy for inflammatory bowel diseases. *Gastroenterology, 152*(2), 398–414.

Lewis, J. D., Sandler, R. S., Brotherton, C., Brensinger, C., Li, H., Kappelman, M. D., Daniel, S. G., Bittinger, K., Albenberg, L., Valentine, J. F., Hanson, J. S., Suskind, D. L., Meyer, A., Compher, C. W., Bewtra, M., Saxena, A., Dobes, A., Cohen, B. L., Flynn, A. D., Fischer, M., Saha, S., Swaminath, A., Yacyshyn, B., Scherl, E., Horst, S., Curtis, J. R., Braly, K., Nessel, L., McCauley, M., McKeever, L. & Herfarth, H.; DINE-CD Study Group. (2021). A randomized trial comparing the specific carbohydrate diet to a Mediterranean diet in adults with Crohn's disease. *Gastroenterology, 161*(3), 837–852.

Mahadevan, U., McConnell, R. A. & Chambers, C. D. (2017). Drug safety and risk of adverse outcomes for pregnant patients with inflammatory bowel disease. *Gastroenterology, 152*(2), 451–462.

Navarro Llavat, M., García-Bosch, O., Castro-Poceiro, J., Bargalló García, A., Ruiz Arroyo, D., Navas Bravo, Y., ... & Domènech Morral, E. (2023). P513 Prospective study on patients' satisfaction and impact on quality of life of corticosteroid therapy in patients with Inflammatory Bowel Disease. *Journal of Crohn's and Colitis, 17*(Supplement_1), i642–i642.

Peng, Z., Yi, J. & Liu, X. (2022). A low-FODMAP diet provides benefits for functional gastrointestinal symptoms but not for improving stool consistency and mucosal inflammation in IBD: a systematic review and meta-analysis. *Nutrients*, 14(10), 2072.

Sasson, A. N., Ananthakrishnan, A. N. & Raman, M. (2021). Diet in treatment of inflammatory bowel diseases. *Clinical Gastroenterology and Hepatology*, 19(3), 425–435.

Shafiee, N. H., Manaf, Z. A., Mokhtar, N. M. & Ali, R. A. R. (2021). Anti-inflammatory diet and inflammatory bowel disease: what clinicians and patients should know? *Intestinal research*, 19(2), 171–185.

Shivaji, U. N., Sharratt, C. L., Thomas, T., Smith, S. C., Iacucci, M., Moran, G. W., Ghosh, S. & Bhala, N. (2019). Managing the adverse events caused by anti-TNF therapy in inflammatory bowel disease. *Alimentary Pharmacology & Therapeutics*, 49(6), 664–680.

Suskind, D. L., Wahbeh, G., Cohen, S. A., Damman, C. J., Klein, J., Braly, K., Shaffer, M. & Lee, D. (2016). Patients perceive clinical benefit with the specific carbohydrate diet for inflammatory bowel disease. *Digestive Diseases and Sciences*, 61, 3255–3260.

Waljee, A. K., Wiitala, W. L., Govani, S., Stidham, R., Saini, S., Hou, J., Feagins, L. A., Khan, N., Good, C. B., Vijan, S. & Higgins, P. D. (2016). Corticosteroid use and complications in a US inflammatory bowel disease cohort. *PLoS One*, 11(6), e0158017.

Wong, D. J., Roth, E. M., Feuerstein, J. D. & Poylin, V. Y. (2019). Surgery in the age of biologics, *Gastroenterology Report*, 7(2), 77–90.

Zhan, Y. A. & Dai, S. X. (2018). Is a low FODMAP diet beneficial for patients with inflammatory bowel disease? A meta-analysis and systematic review. *Clinical Nutrition*, 37(1), 123–129.

Part II

Psychotherapy for Patients with IBD

Common Psychiatric Comorbidities

4

Given the complexities of living with an IBD, it is not surprising that rates of psychiatric comorbidity in patients with IBD (and especially in patients with secondary IBS) are significantly higher than in healthy controls—typically around 40%. Common comorbid psychiatric diagnoses include ARFID, panic disorder, agoraphobia, illness anxiety, social anxiety, OCD, PTSD, and major depression. Unsurprisingly, psychiatric comorbidity is related to disease severity and physical comorbidities. The greater the burden of disease, the more likely it is to affect emotional and mental health. But this also works in the other direction—greater distress and maladaptive coping can adversely affect physical health as well. Psychiatric comorbidity is also associated with lower health related quality of life and higher rates of medical or health care utilization, as well as higher perceived symptom burden. Alarmingly, psychiatric comorbidity is even associated with higher rates of mortality in patients with a range of immune-mediated diseases, including IBD. Thus, identifying and addressing psychiatric comorbidity in patients with IBD is incredibly important. Fortunately, CBT therapists are well trained to do exactly this.

Now that you know a lot more about the challenges of living with and managing an IBD, we will turn to the role of CBT in helping IBD patients achieve the best possible quality of life. This treatment manual assumes good working knowledge of a number of core CBT principles and techniques for the treatment of depression, panic and agoraphobia, health anxiety, social anxiety, obsessive-compulsive disorder, and post-traumatic stress disorder. What follows in this chapter is a description of the most common psychiatric comorbidities and problems you are likely to encounter in patients with IBD,

DOI: 10.4324/9781003454380-7

along with guidance on how to apply (and sometimes adapt) standard CBT treatments to this population.

Fear of Food and Avoidant Restrictive Food Intake Disorder (ARFID)

ARFID is one of the most common diagnoses we tend to see in patients with chronic GI disorders. Recall that the scientific evidence for the benefits of highly restrictive diets in IBD is quite limited, but there are a lot of diets out there that purport to reduce inflammation and/or to help control symptoms by restricting specific foods. It is hard not to believe that, when you are suffering from a chronic digestive disorder, what you eat must matter. That's common sense. And there are some dietary adjustments that some patients with IBD will absolutely need to make (like avoiding high residue foods or limiting insoluble fiber). However, restricting one food or group of foods can quickly turn into restricting lots of different foods. If someone's diet has become so restricted that it is causing interference (either secondary to malnutrition and/or to significant social and emotional distress or dysfunction) then the person may well meet criteria for ARFID. Fear of food can contribute significantly to reduced quality of life, social impairment, and anxiety.

ARFID comes in two basic subtypes—extreme picky eating and fear based. Picky eaters typically *dislike* whole categories of food and find them distasteful or even actively disgusting. Fear based ARFID, in which the patient avoids whole categories of foods for fear of negative consequences, is quite different from extreme picky eating. Patients with fear based ARFID, in contrast, still like foods and *wish* they could eat them, but are terrified of experiencing adverse effects, including GI symptoms like choking, nausea, vomiting, pain, urgent diarrhea, or bowel obstructions. Interestingly, most of the dietary plans for IBD (including the low residue diet, the IBD Anti-Inflammatory Diet, and the Low FODMAP Diet) all strongly recommend reintroduction of restricted foods to achieve the least restrictive diet possible. Malnutrition and nutrient malabsorption are significant problems for IBD patients, and eating as varied, wholesome, and nutritious a diet as possible is the best way to offset this. Only the Specific Carbohydrate Diet recommends life long abstention from the restricted grains and potatoes. Despite this, many patients with IBD are afraid to reintroduce avoided foods. Some are even terrified.

Given the degree to which socializing, family events, cultural and ethnic identity and hedonic pleasure in life all revolve around food, it is easy to see why significant fear of food can be truly life impairing. If the patient meets criteria for ARFID, addressing this in therapy (perhaps in collaboration with a good dietician if you and the patient are lucky enough to find one to work with) is important.

ARFID is best conceptualized as an example of *maladaptive avoidance.* Like any other avoidance behavior, the best approach is a combination of cognitive therapy (*de-catastrophizing*) followed with *exposure therapy.* But as with many things in IBD, you do need to ensure that the patient's fear of food is actually maladaptive. Thus, before you diagnose and treat ARFID, you need to try to determine the degree to which their restrictive diet is actually medically warranted. If the patient has a dietician, you should absolutely consult with that individual. In the more likely situation in which the patient does not have access to a dietician, then you should consult with the patient's gastroenterologist. Although most GI docs don't get a lot of training in nutrition, they can certainly comment on the medical necessity of certain dietary restrictions. This is especially important if the patient has existing strictures or a history of bowel obstructions. They may truly need to avoid foods that are highly fibrous, chunky, sharp, or very high in insoluble fiber. In this case, the patient may need help addressing their own frustration or embarrassment with needing to eat a "weird" diet. In that case, you should pivot to addressing anger, sadness, and social anxiety.

Sometimes patients avoid socializing or eating out because it feels too embarrassing to "explain" why they have so many restrictions. Patients are often sure that waiters will be annoyed with them, or that other people will perceive them as needy or whiny or demanding. Patients often fear being judged negatively in some way by others. It can be important to reframe this—most restaurants now routinely ask about allergies and other restrictions like gluten for celiac patients. Suggest that the patient try some experiments of going out to eat and asking the server about specific dishes or ingredients. A few servers may seem impatient, but the vast majority will simply take this in stride.

Patients often worry about what family, friends, or colleagues will think, both at restaurants, or if they are invited to someone's home for a meal. They don't want to be perceived as a prima donna who is demanding and difficult. They also don't want people to feel sorry for them. Suggest perspective taking—if the patient invited a friend over for dinner and the friend told them they were deathly allergic to legumes or shellfish, or had celiac disease, surely the patient would be gracious and would do their best to accommodate their friend's dietary restrictions without thinking twice about it. Why would the patient deny their own friends the opportunity to do that for them? Treat this as you would any other social anxiety. Do some cognitive reappraisal and set up some easy exposures and behavioral experiments. You should certainly encourage your patient to go out with people, even if they have to eat a small, safe meal beforehand. Going to a restaurant and ordering a small cup of broth while their friend eats a full meal may feel "weird" but it is more important to spend time with friends than to avoid potential embarrassment when the waiter asks yet again if they can get you something. Treat this like any other exposure exercise.

Taking an Acceptance Therapy approach can be useful here as well. Ask the patient to clarify what their *values* are around shared meal times and social-izing. Many people will point to the importance of company, shared conversation, and opportunities for both fun and intimacy. They may even share how much they miss normal socializing. The food itself and what people do (or don't) eat may not even be that important. They may also realize that it is important to them not to "burden" other people with catering to their needs. On the other hand they may worry about insulting a cook by not eating what is put in front of them, or picking at their food. In some families, refusing Grandma's special recipe or not taking seconds that are urged upon one is thought to be rude and can cause family conflict. Sometimes a good first step is to have them invite people to their own home for a meal. That way they have total control over the menu, but can still provide for others and enjoy the evening. Alternatively, encouraging people to be honest with family and friends is often the best approach. Surely Grandma wouldn't *want* them to eat her special holiday fill-in-the-blank if she knew it was going to make them ill. The overall approach here, if the patient does indeed need to follow a fairly restrictive diet, is to target the cognitive distortions and maladaptive avoidance that underlie the anxiety about eating with others.

On the other hand, if the patient eats a highly restricted diet that is *not* medically warranted, then they may well meet criteria for ARFID and you will need to use CBT skills to get them to reintroduce feared foods. In other words, you want them to try to expand their diet to be the least restrictive version possible. Recall that almost all the IBD specific diets and the Low FODMAP Diet typically encourage systematic reintroduction of the restricted foods after an initial strict elimination phase. If a stray onion or some dairy or wheat should find its way into a meal they are served, it won't be the end of the world.

Treatment for ARFID is typically going to feel just like treatment for specific phobia. Encourage the patient to construct a hierarchy of feared foods, and then tackle the one that feels the easiest. Then slowly work your way up the hierarchy, tackling small servings first and then slightly larger ones. If the patient has difficulty deciding which food to try, ask them what they miss the most. This will sometimes help clarify the order in which they want to reintroduce foods. I had one patient who was absolutely terrified of yogurt. Both her dietician and I kept encouraging her to try some—even just a teaspoon! It took a month for her to muster the courage to try it. When nothing bad happened, she was brave enough to try a slightly larger serving. Today she happily eats four to six ounces of yogurt most days with breakfast and enjoys it very much. It's probably really good for her microbiome, and certainly hasn't increased her inflammation or GI symptoms.

ARFID can also be secondary to PTSD related to prior medical emergencies like bowel obstructions or severe pain and bloody stool. If the person's IBD has improved—either through medication or surgery—and their doctor approves a more varied diet, they may still be afraid of trying a food that previously led to an obstruction or caused them significant pain and bloody diarrhea. This is completely understandable, and needs empathy and understanding. Just as with PTSD, however, it may be that the food *was* dangerous at the time, but is no longer dangerous to them. Continuing to avoid the food simply perpetuates the fear. Start by having the patient recount the events that led them to fear the food in the first place. It may simply be that they were so symptomatic at some point that eating just about *anything* exacerbated their symptoms. If they are medically more stable now, they will have to be brave and start experimenting with a more varied diet again.

At its most extreme, some patients refuse to eat *anything* other than pureed foods, baby foods or blended liquid smoothies and meal replacements. In the vast majority of cases, this is not appropriate or warranted, and is truly limiting nutritionally, socially, and hedonically. After getting the okay from the patient's doctor, you should plan an exposure hierarchy with the patient to start reintroducing semi-solid and then solid food back into their diet. If they are reluctant, I often encourage them to think back on when they enjoyed eating "real" food. What food do they miss the most? Getting them to list the foods they most hunger for can be a good way to motivate patients to overcome their fear. As with all exposure therapy exercises, work with the patient collaboratively to come up with the assignments, and be sure the patient understands the rationale for why you are encouraging them to eat a more varied diet.

A caveat to this is that if the patient is maintaining their weight and nutritional status on a mostly or even fully liquid diet, their IBD is under good control, and they are not distressed or limited by this, then they probably *don't* meet criteria for ARFID. They may tell you that they are very content. Grabbing a Ka'Chava smoothie in the morning, a Kate Farms shake for lunch, and a pureed soup for dinner is convenient, nutritious, and doesn't negatively impact their social life. Some patients with gastroparesis (a motility disorder in which the stomach cannot push solid food into the small intestine) settle on this approach, and after an initial adjustment period are perfectly well adjusted socially and emotionally. The upshot is that you should treat fear of food if it is indeed causing distress and impairment, but as always, a thorough evaluation with each individual patient is crucial.

Panic Disorder and Agoraphobia

Panic disorder, and even more importantly, agoraphobia, are very common comorbidities in IBD. The cognitive model of panic suggests that people engage in catastrophic misinterpretations of (basically benign) body sensations. Unfortunately, people with IBD have lots of body sensations that may, or may well not, be benign. It's really easy for patients to assume that every gas bubble, twinge, or loose stool signifies an uptick in inflammation, or lack of response to medication and worsening disease. Even if the patient has never experienced an obstruction, they may constantly scan their body for signs that they might be experiencing one. Sometimes it is hard for a patient with IBD to remember that everyone experiences GI discomfort from time to time. Assuming their IBD is under good medical control, they can probably safely ignore most of the little sensations they experience day to day. It certainly isn't helpful to catastrophize them and get terribly anxious about the possibility of escalating illness. Finding the right balance between appropriate surveillance of symptoms that might suggest increasing inflammation, and learning to ignore lots of little uninformative discomfort signals is important in helping people not panic.

Agoraphobia in IBD patients is much more common than pure panic disorder, and may not be associated with true panic at all, or at least not full symptom panic attacks. Rather, people may become very anxious about being too far away from a bathroom, or about experiencing urgency or severe abdominal pain when they are away from home. Sometimes referred to as bowel control anxiety, or fear of fecal incontinence (FI), this sub-type of agoraphobia is specific to people with GI disorders. Some patients simply take urgency and frequency in stride. They have no problem stopping at random restaurants or gas stations or asking store managers to use the restroom even in places where it isn't normally available. They always pack a change of clothes and some wipes in their car or bag "just in case," and don't let their IBD stop them from living their lives fully. Other people become very anxious about being caught out and worry a great deal about inconveniencing others, embarrassing themselves, occupying public restrooms for lengthy periods of time, or worst yet soiling themselves in public. Alas, for many patients with IBD, this is *not* a catastrophic distortion. Many folks with IBD have actually experienced fecal incontinence at some point in their life.

Fear of FI can underlie or dramatically exacerbate agoraphobia, social anxiety, PTSD, and depression. With the advent of DSM-5, fear of fecal incontinence is a sufficient underlying motivation for a diagnosis of agoraphobia. It is worth asking patients if they have ever actually experienced one (or more) episodes of FI. FI is unfortunately not uncommon in IBD patients (approximately one in four patients or 24% have experienced at least one lifetime episode). FI is associated with significant emotional distress, disability, and avoidance. Unfortunately, less than half of patients with FI actually talk to their gastroenterologist about it, and even fewer seek treatment or are aware that there are specialists in this area and interventions that can be quite helpful. For example, pelvic floor physical therapists who specialize in incontinence can provide biofeedback training that can be quite effective. Other interventions include surgery and nerve stimulation procedures that can retrain the anal sphincter and the rectum to work in concert to retain stool until the patient is ready to go. Patients with secondary IBS may be even more likely to have experienced at least one episode of FI. If the IBD is actually in remission but they are still experiencing urgency secondary to IBS, then teaching them to use deep diaphragmatic breathing (DDB) to "hold it" or delay defecation even when they are feeling cramping, can be enormously helpful.

Fear of FI can cause a good deal of maladaptive avoidance and can contribute to both agoraphobia and social anxiety. Many patients will avoid places where a bathroom might be far away (beaches, parks, sport tournaments on large fields, concert venues) or where there might be long lines or where the bathroom might be occupied or embarrassing to "stink up" or occupy for a long period of time (e.g., restaurants). Fear of FI can also contribute to social isolation, relationship issues, and depression. Some patients are terrified of experiencing FI around potential sexual partners or even around friends or complete strangers. The avoidance of social venues, outings, and get-togethers can lead to loneliness and hopelessness about ever being able to have a full and normal life. Some patients are convinced that no one could ever love them if they knew about their IBD.

It is easy for a therapist to have empathy with this fear, but it is important not to shy away from both exposure therapy (to reduce avoidance) and de-catastrophizing and cognitive reappraisal. Exposure therapy mostly consists of encouraging the person to *go* to places and do things they have been avoiding. This could mean going for walks, taking public transportation, going to concerts or sporting events, or out to dinner with friends. They can certainly practice requesting to use the restroom at stores and other places (e.g., banks, pharmacies, eyeglass repair shops) that do not normally have public restrooms available. Most states have laws mandating that businesses make restrooms available to the public in case of medical necessity. (This is typically referred to as Ally's Law, in honor of a young teenager with Crohn's who did soil herself while out shopping with her mother. Her mother lobbied her state legislature and succeeded in getting the first of these laws passed.) Patients may have to overcome significant social anxiety to even request this, and may need help interpreting the data they collect appropriately. For example, a lower level employee at a stationary store may feel it is above their pay grade to allow someone in the back to use the staff bathroom, but may suggest the shoe store two doors down. This doesn't mean the person was annoyed or that the request was unreasonable or inappropriate.

The Crohn's and Colitis Foundation (CCF) will also provide patients with Washroom Access Cards that can be used to help demonstrate medical necessity. There are also apps available that will help patients locate usable public restrooms (and will sometimes crowdsource ratings of the restrooms as well with respect to cleanliness). The We Can't Wait app, developed by the CCF, is a good example. Unfortunately, these apps don't always have enough information about specific locations, so they're not always super useful. But in some places (especially in more urban areas) they can be quite helpful.

If the patient has actually experienced incontinence, it may be reasonable for them to use anti-diarrheal agents prior to outings where bathrooms may be difficult to access. It is also important to think through how to manage it if the patient actually does experience incontinence. For example, it might be reasonable to keep a change of clothes and some wet wipes in the car or in a day pack. While such contingency planning might be considered maladaptive safety seeking behavior in IBS, in IBD patients it might simply be appropriate problem solving, and having a "go bag" at the ready during outings can provide significant reassurance in the event that they do have an accident.

One thing I would *not* recommend is *in vivo* exposure therapy with actual poop. Folks who are anxious about sweating might well be encouraged to spray their underarms and faces with water and then go to the mall and walk around. Putting real or even fake poop in your underwear and walking around the mall is not a good idea. Poop is gross. It smells. It's dirty. It's not good for your skin to be in contact with it. It is universally taboo in every human culture. But you *can* encourage your patient to go to the mall and walk around even on a day when they're not feeling great. Practice being in a store and then asking for access to the nearest washroom to deal with an urgent medical need.

Patients can be encouraged to voice their catastrophic fears and to de-catastrophize. Yes, soiling yourself would be highly inconvenient and potentially quite embarrassing. But even if it happened, it need not be the end of the world. They can probably discreetly retire to clean up. Many people might not even notice. Even if someone did notice, the vast majority of people are kind and understanding, and would either pretend to ignore it, or would offer to help. Imaginal exposure and planful problem solving can be quite useful here.

Health Anxiety

Many people with health anxiety (up to and including illness anxiety disorder) don't really have any serious underlying physical conditions at all. They may feel very anxious and ruminate a lot about possible illnesses. They may seek reassurance or go to lots of doctors or spend a lot of time googling various physical signs and symptoms trying to figure out if that red spot on their arm is skin cancer or whether feeling lightheaded and bumping into a chair is a sign of impending multiple sclerosis. But people who have genuine underlying chronic conditions like IBD may also suffer from health anxiety. This can take two basic forms: worry about the underlying disease itself and worry about possible adverse effects of medications. The tricky thing is that sometimes physical signs and symptoms really DO signal something that needs attention. For example, patients on many IBD specific immunosuppressive drugs really are at greater risk for skin cancer, so noticing new weird spots on their skin (especially on the face or along the hairline) might actually be important. But there is a difference between appropriate surveillance, along with yearly trips to a dermatologist, and daily scrutiny of every possible skin tag, mole, freckle, and cherry angioma, along with spikes in anxiety every time they think they see something that might be new. Helping patients learn to discriminate between pain that signals something urgent (say a sudden abdominal pain that stops them in their tracks, makes them catch their breath and bend over, and doesn't resolve for 30 minutes) and discomfort that can be safely ignored (some gurgling and gas pain that recedes as soon as they fart or poop) can be important. This can dramatically decrease unnecessary medical utilization and especially unhelpful emergency room visits.

Social Anxiety Disorder

Shame and secrecy are very common problems for patients with IBD. Remember that gut issues and poop really are taboo subjects in pretty much every culture in the world. Many patients with IBD worry about being humiliated or embarrassed by a number of aspects of their disease, from gut noises and frequent bathroom trips up to and including fecal incontinence. They also worry about people finding them disgusting. Many folks try hard to keep their IBD secret, which can lead to a good deal of social anxiety. Shame and secrecy get in the way of true emotional intimacy and often contribute to low self-esteem or even to core defectiveness schemas that can drive significant depression. Yes, poop is yucky and taboo, but you should help your patient find ways to talk about their IBD in factual, confident terms. There is considerable evidence that keeping GI issues secret, especially from loved ones, is strongly associated with poor relationship satisfaction and lower well-being.

Social anxiety can be triggered by quite a few aspects of IBD and is almost always related to cognitive distortions about what other people are thinking. For example, someone might be terribly embarrassed about going to a restaurant and needing to order odd food, or to eat very little. Alternatively they might not have a problem with the food itself, but might be very anxious about the possibility that they will need to excuse themselves from the table to use the bathroom. In both cases, they might be worrying about how other people are interpreting their behavior. Like all humans, patients with IBD are vulnerable to the spotlight effect, in which they think their behavior really stands out and is being scrutinized (and judged) by others far more than it actually is. People need help identifying those cognitive distortions and recognizing them as such. They may also need help setting up exposures and behavioral experiments to convince themselves that being honest about their issues won't expose them to censure, ridicule or disgust. I met one patient at an IBD support group who had never shared the fact that she had chronic GI issues with anyone at the office, and often felt trapped in meetings and terrified of her issues being revealed in any way. She announced unequivocally that if she were ever to experience FI at work, she would pack up her desk and quit immediately and never, ever go back. I think most people would agree that that would be a maladaptive choice based on cognitive distortions about what other people might think. This poor woman lived in fear, and never took the chance to find out whether her co-workers might actually be empathetic and supportive.

If your patient has had surgery, and has scars, or has an ostomy, social anxiety, particularly about dating and sexual intimacy, can be pretty common. I like to tell people that body imperfections are a wonderful litmus test for new partners. If a potential partner is turned off, or worse, is cruel or demeaning, then it is a clear reflection of who that person is, and it definitely puts them in the "do not date this person under any circumstances" column. On the other hand, if the person is tolerant, or better yet tender and curious, then it speaks volumes about their character structure and what it would be like to partner with them. How convenient to have such a useful test available to you!

Some people with IBD just feel broken and damaged and are terrified of revealing any of that to others for fear that it will be reflected back to them. But hiding their disease never gives them the chance to test out whether others will actually view them that way. In many cases, people will actually see them as resilient and brave and strong. As with so many other things, intimacy and trust are only possible when the person is brave enough to show themselves fully, IBD and all. Supporting patients in taking those risks is incredibly important.

Obsessive-Compulsive Disorder

It has been known for many years that OCD and autoimmune disorders have a surprising degree of comorbidity. Some have suggested that OCD itself may be a form of autoimmune reactivity. This is supported in part by the research on pediatric autoimmune neuropsychiatric disorders associated with strepto-coccal infections (PANDAS) which are typically characterized by the sudden onset of OCD and/or tic disorders. There is also evidence that immune-mediated neuroinflammation may underlie OCD in adults, with subgroups of patients with OCD showing elevated proinflammatory cytokines and autoantibodies against neuronal targets including the basal ganglia. From the reverse perspective, there is also data to suggest that OCD in families, espe-cially when there are high levels of contamination obsessions and cleaning compulsions, can increase the risk of autoimmune disorders of various types, including IBD. The "hygiene hypothesis" of autoimmune disorders suggests that over-sterilization of our environment can lead to "dumb" immune systems that cannot distinguish appropriately between harmful invaders and benign proteins, or worse between the harmful invaders and the self. It is easy to see how cleaning compulsions could lead to over-sterilization of the envir-onment! Thus, the overlap between OCD and IBD may be bi-directional, with autoinflammation increasing the risk of OCD, and OCD actually increasing the risk of autoinflammation through excessive cleaning and sterilization of the environment.

Treatment for OCD in patients with IBD, just like treatment for OCD in everyone else, relies on *Exposure and Response Prevention* (ERP). This means the person has to expose themselves to the feared thoughts and situations and stimuli, and then has to resist engaging in the compulsions they would nor-mally do to mitigate their anxiety. Treating OCD in patients with IBD may be complicated, however, by the fact that they often take immunosuppressive medications. A patient on steroids or a biologic drug *is* at increased risk of opportunistic infections, especially upper respiratory and sinus infections. If they wash their hands frequently, carry hand sanitizer with them at all times, and prefer to wear a good mask when out in public, it can be hard to disen-tangle how much of this is perfectly appropriate caution, and how much of it might be driven by underlying OCD. As always, a good case conceptualiza-tion and an understanding of the medical details for your individual patient is important in determining whether this behavior should be a therapeutic target or not.

If a patient of mine presents with OCD, I typically target *other* obsessions and compulsions first. That is, I will prioritize treating obsessions and compulsions that are unrelated to contamination, infection, and cleaning. Typically, as the underlying OCD "circuit" starts to calm down, the patient will often come to realize that some of their behavior related to infection control and hygiene, or disease management, is excessive and unnecessary. For example, I had one patient with moderate OCD and Crohn's who continued to wear gloves, carry hand sanitizer, avoid large public venues and wear a mask whenever in public long after the vast majority of people had been vaccinated for COVID and relaxed their infection control. She believed this behavior was essential to protect her from devastating infection. Instead of tackling this head on, we worked on *other* aspects of her OCD, such as her obsessions about harm coming to her adult children, or one of them becoming suicidal or unemployed or remaining single forever because she had said or done the wrong thing. (Of note, both her children, though single, were highly successful in their respective careers and seemed perfectly well adjusted and healthy.) Once she finally dropped the compulsion of saying "God forbid!" every time we did exposure therapy on this, she made good progress on all of her OCD related content, including the infection control compulsions.

Some patients with IBD may develop elaborate rituals around cleaning themselves after pooping. This may be particularly heartbreaking in women with rectal–vaginal fistulas. They may be constantly concerned about leaking stool and may worry a great deal about foul odors or staining their clothes. This is *not* OCD and should be treated with compassion and validation. As always, a thorough assessment, and really understanding what is necessary in order to manage the IBD, versus what is excessive and interfering, is crucial, and is helped by good working knowledge of IBD itself.

Post-Traumatic Stress Disorder

Many IBD patients have experienced trauma of some sort in the course of managing their illness. Maybe they experienced a humiliating episode of fecal incontinence. Maybe they had to undergo nocturnal enteral feeding as a kid and never got to go to sleepovers or to summer camp as a result. Maybe they had a small bowel obstruction that was misdiagnosed by a tired, dismissive ER doctor and then turned into a life-threatening emergency. Maybe a gastroenterologist early on jumped too quickly to suggesting a radical colectomy and permanent ostomy, leaving a young patient terrified and hopeless about ever having a "normal" life. Maybe they suffered from sepsis after surgery and spent months recovering after a lengthy ICU stay. Of course, patients with IBD may also have trauma histories that are completely unrelated to their IBD.

Such stories will often emerge during a thorough history in the first few sessions, but may not emerge until later in therapy when the patient trusts the therapist enough to talk about it. As with most trauma, simply telling the story and letting themselves relive the emotions of the time can be enormously therapeutic. Sometimes writing about the trauma just once outside of session, and then reading the narrative to the therapist is enough. Sometimes writing a "letter" (that they don't send), to a provider who let them down or a gas station attendant who refused to give them access to the restroom, expressing their anger and frustration can be helpful. Sometimes writing a letter to their younger self, or utilizing an "empty chair" technique in which they imagine talking to their younger self there in the office, offering words of encouragement and perspective, can feel very therapeutic. Here is where a creative therapist, who is knowledgeable about trauma treatment generally, can be very helpful. One does not typically need to do a full Prolonged Exposure (PE), Cognitive Processing Therapy (CPT) or Eye Movement Desensitization and Reprocessing (EMDR) protocol to get a good therapeutic response. Sometimes just giving the patient space to tell the story is enough. This relies on the transdiagnostic principle that exposure to previously avoided anxiety-provoking material often leads to both reinterpretation and habituation. Of course, if a therapist is knowledgeable about various empirically supported approaches to trauma, bringing in components of PE, CPT, EMDR, or Imaginal Rescripting may indeed be warranted or even necessary. I encourage therapists to utilize whichever evidence based approach to trauma they are most comfortable with.

Depression

There is considerable evidence that IBD and depression often co-occur. The direction of causality remains unclear, but it is likely that the links are bi-directional. As with OCD, there is some evidence that the inflammatory cytokines, HPA axis dysregulation, microbiome disturbances, and immune dysregulation of IBD may contribute directly to disorders of central nervous system dysregulation, including depression. There is no question that dealing with a chronic, sometimes debilitating, occasionally frightening disease takes a toll on people and can set the stage for hopelessness and helplessness about the self and the future. Depression, in turn, can make it more difficult for patients with IBD to cope proactively. Medication adherence, eating healthfully, and staying physically active, all of which are important aspects of disease management, are all much harder when the patient is depressed. In particular, the fatigue that often goes hand in hand with IBD can make it difficult for people to sustain motivation and remain engaged in work, love, and play. Withdrawal from life's activities secondary to fatigue, or pain, or bowel control anxiety can contribute to the start of a depressive episode, or can exacerbate any underlying depression that was already there. Gentle behavioral activation is always a good first line approach with these folks.

Addressing depression in a patient with IBD requires a thorough understanding of their history and their prognosis. Patients who are newly diagnosed may be feeling overwhelmed, frightened, and hopeless. Helping patients understand that most people respond fairly well to treatment, and that there is no reason to think they will not be able to lead a full, normal life can be incredibly important. Their doctor may have tried to convey this, or may think they did, but any such reassurance often gets lost in those initial medical appointments that go by very quickly and typically focus on discussing test results and recommending treatments.

Patients who have been living with IBD for some time may feel very demoralized if their disease has progressed despite active treatment. Faced with the need for surgery, or switching to a drug with a more anxiety provoking list of adverse effects can make people feel afraid and hopeless about their future. New fistulas, or the onset of related symptoms like rheumatoid pain in the hands, can be overwhelming and incredibly frustrating. Addressing any cognitive distortions or catastrophizing can often be helpful. But sometimes, as even the late, great Dr. Aaron T. Beck used to say, you just have to be there with the patient and empathize with their pain.

Despite the many real challenges of living with an IBD, I often find that the tried and true cognitive therapy techniques, like filling out thought records, cognitive reappraisal, and schema work to get at underlying core beliefs can be incredibly helpful. People often don't question their negative automatic thoughts or their catastrophic beliefs. They may well be entertaining negative thoughts like "There's no point in trying to go for a walk. I'll just feel terrible afterwards," or extreme thoughts like "No one will ever love me once they learn about this," or "life won't be worth living if I can't eat normally," or "I'll probably be the person who gets all the horrible side effects and I'll end up dying of cancer." Identifying those beliefs, understanding the impact they have on mood, and then addressing them by coming up with benign alternatives and examining the evidence for and against them works just as well for patients with IBD as it does for other depressed patients. Many people with an IBD assume that physical activity will make them feel worse. In fact, gentle physical activity and exercise have anti-inflammatory effects and can make people feel better. Introduce your patient to the concept of *behavioral experiments* and see if they will agree to try something out, acknowledging that you take a scientific approach to all this, and you'll be open to being proved wrong. A combination of behavioral activation, better diet, and cognitive reappraisal can work wonders for many depressed patients.

Anyone who has worked with depressed patients knows that sometimes hopelessness can lead to suicidality. You should always be alert to statements indicating that the patient may be feeling suicidal or experiencing passive suicidal ideation. "I don't know if I can do this anymore." "I can't go on like this." "Life just isn't fun with this disease." "What's the point in trying a new medicine? It'll just fail like all the others." "If this doesn't work, I don't know what I'll do." Or the scariest thing a patient can say: "I'm such a burden. My family would be better off without me." The wise therapist will immediately call attention to such statements and ask the patient to elaborate. You should never shy away from asking the patient directly if they are thinking about hurting themselves or wishing they were dead. Every experienced therapist should know how to do a risk evaluation, and to intervene effectively and immediately. Ask "Has it gotten so bad that you think about hurting yourself or trying to end your life?" Many patients will endorse passive suicidal ideation, but will adamantly deny intent or any plan. Most will say "I would never actually do anything to hurt myself" and will spontaneously share reasons for not dying like "I could never do that to my family."

If your patient is experiencing active suicidal ideation, however, you will need to intervene more directly. As always, assess intent and access to means. Review reasons for living *and* reasons for not dying. Acknowledge the real challenges and pain of living with an IBD, but guide the patient to develop a safety plan. With the patient's consent, pull in people from their support system—partners, family, friends. Have them call someone right there and then to be sure they won't be going home to an empty house or apartment. Have them get a trusted someone to hide the medication or remove the gun or ammunition from the home. I reserve hospitalization only for those patients who cannot commit to a safety plan, to disposing of or securing means, and are not sure themselves whether they will be safe at home. I much prefer to manage suicidality on an outpatient basis whenever possible, and I have never actually recommended hospitalization for any of my patients with

IBD (although I have done so with other patients on rare occasions). That said, hospitalization can be lifesaving for some patients, and if you are truly worried about your patient's safety, then talk to them about the possibility of a brief inpatient stay.

Ideally, you will be able to help inspire hope. It can be very helpful to remind patients that IBD tend to wax and wane. They may be very fatigued and in pain today, but there is a very good chance that the flare they are in will remit and they will feel much better again. You should always ensure that the patient is communicating effectively with their gastroenterologist. Indeed, this is a good time to reach out to the GI doc to ensure that you understand the patient's treatment plan and prognosis yourself. The doctor may well be able to share that they have a plan B, C, and D if the patient does not respond well to the current management plan. Remind patients that while suicide would end their current pain, it also guarantees that they will *never* feel joy or love or satisfaction or pleasure in the future. It also guarantees their loved ones a lifetime of remorse, pain, and anger, and increases the risk of suicide for everyone else in their family system. Suicide is a solution to intolerable pain. But it's a *terrible* solution. Help the patient have hope for better days ahead.

In the rare cases in which the person's IBD is truly out of control, sometimes all you can do is help the patient find meaning and purpose in the life that they do have available to them. Very occasionally, you will meet a patient with a history of poor response to multiple medications, several failed surgeries, short bowel syndrome from numerous resections, chronic, painful fistulas or pouchitis that just won't resolve. They may be truly disabled and unable to work or complete schooling. This is a tough road for some patients, and inappropriate optimism can feel invalidating to them. On the other hand, helping the patient identify which aspects of life they *can* still enjoy and take part in can certainly be therapeutic. Like anyone with a chronic or debilitating condition, there are still moments of grace and joy and connection that can make life worth living. Help the patient identify what brings about those moments for them.

I like to remind people that new drugs are being developed every day, often targeting newly discovered mechanisms. If they can hold on, there is a chance that they will indeed get relief in the future. Participating in research opportunities through CCF initiatives like IBD Qorus and SPARC IBD (Study of a Prospective Adult Research Cohort with IBD) can give people a sense of purpose. These are very large, multi-site research initiatives that combine data from thousands of IBD patients around the country. The team leaders centralize and link data from diverse research studies to facilitate sharing across the research community. Stakeholder feedback and patient perspectives are always included. Even if their own IBD isn't under control, they can contribute to the growing body of knowledge that may well benefit all IBD patients down the road.

Despite the possibility that you will encounter a patient with severe or suicidal depression, be assured that the vast majority of patients with IBD will experience only transient, mild, or moderate depressive symptoms that typically respond quite well to standard CBT techniques. Being knowledgeable about the real challenges they face can be very helpful, but don't hesitate to challenge cognitive distortions, encourage behavioral activation, use motivational interviewing to get them off the couch, set up behavioral experiments to help them learn that people will still respect and love them and that they can lead full, rich lives even with their IBD in the background.

Summary

Patients with IBD are at increased risk for a number of psychiatric comorbidities, including ARFID, panic and agoraphobia, illness anxiety, social anxiety, OCD, PTSD, and depression. Hopefully you now have a better understanding of how IBD specific content may underlie or exacerbate each disorder. Experienced cognitive behavioral therapists will be very familiar with a range of CBT protocols, techniques, procedures, and evidence based practices that can be brought to bear to treat each comorbidity in the context of IBD. The chapter assumed a fair degree of familiarity with a range of CBT interventions, including thought records, cognitive reappraisal and de-catastrophizing, exposure therapy and behavioral experiments, as well as knowledge of some specific CBT protocols, such as Exposure and Response Prevention (ERP), Prolonged Exposure (PE), Cognitive Processing Therapy (CPT), Eye Movement Desensitization and Reprocessing (EMDR) or Imaginal Rescripting for trauma. Experienced and creative therapists should be able to adapt all of these to include IBD specific material and modifications in ways that will make the therapy far more effective and will help patients with IBD lead richer, more satisfying lives. Addressing psychiatric comorbidity can go a long way to reducing distress and disability in patients with IBD.

Bibliography

Abautret-Daly, Á., Dempsey, E., Parra-Blanco, A., Medina, C. & Harkin, A. (2018). Gut–brain actions underlying comorbid anxiety and depression associated with inflammatory bowel disease. *Acta Neuropsychiatrica, 30*(5), 275–296.

Bannaga, A. S. & Selinger, C. P. (2015). Inflammatory bowel disease and anxiety: links, risks, and challenges faced. *Clinical and Experimental Gastroenterology*, 111–117.

Barberio, B., Zamani, M., Black, C. J., Savarino, E. V. & Ford, A. C. (2021). Prevalence of symptoms of anxiety and depression in patients with inflammatory bowel disease: a systematic review and meta-analysis. *The Lancet Gastroenterology & Hepatology, 6*(5), 359–370.

Bernstein, C. N., Hitchon, C. A., Walld, R., Bolton, J. M., Lix, L. M., El-Gabalawy, R., ... & Marrie, R. A. (2021). The impact of psychiatric comorbidity on health care utilization in inflammatory bowel disease: a population-based study. *Inflammatory Bowel Diseases, 27*(9), 1462–1474.

Bisgaard, T. H., Allin, K. H., Keefer, L., Ananthakrishnan, A. N. & Jess, T. (2022). Depression and anxiety in inflammatory bowel disease: epidemiology, mechanisms and treatment. *Nature Reviews Gastroenterology & Hepatology, 19*(11), 717–726.

Filipovic, B. R. & Filipovic, B. F. (2014). Psychiatric comorbidity in the treatment of patients with inflammatory bowel disease. *World Journal of Gastroenterology: WJG, 20*(13), 3552.

Fink, M., Simons, M., Tomasino, K., Pandit, A. & Taft, T. (2022). When is patient behavior indicative of avoidant restrictive food intake disorder (ARFID) vs reasonable response to digestive disease? *Clinical Gastroenterology and Hepatology, 20*(6), 1241–1250.

Guo, L., Rohde, J. & Farraye, F. A. (2020). Stigma and disclosure in patients with inflammatory bowel disease. *Inflammatory Bowel Diseases, 26*(7), 1010–1016.

Hu, S., Chen, Y., Chen, Y. & Wang, C. (2021). Depression and anxiety disorders in patients with inflammatory bowel disease. *Frontiers in Psychiatry, 12*, 714057.

Lenti, M. V., Cococcia, S., Ghorayeb, J., Di Sabatino, A. & Selinger, C. P. (2020). Stigmatisation and resilience in inflammatory bowel disease. *Internal and Emergency Medicine, 15*, 211–223.

Marrie, R. A., Walld, R., Bolton, J. M., Sareen, J., Patten, S. B., Singer, A., Lix, L. M., Hitchon, C. A., El-Gabalawy, R., Katz, A., Risk, J. D. & Bernstein, C. N. (2018). Psychiatric comorbidity increases mortality in immune-mediated inflammatory diseases. *General Hospital Psychiatry, 53*, 65–72.

Marrie, R. A., Walld, R., Bolton, J. M., Sareen, J., Walker, J. R., Patten, S. B., Singer, A., Lix, L. M., Hitchon, C., A., El-Gabalawy, R., Katz, A., Fisk, J. D. & Bernstein,

C. N. (2018). Physical comorbidities increase the risk of psychiatric comorbidity in immune-mediated inflammatory disease. *General Hospital Psychiatry, 51*, 71–78.

Mikocka-Walus, A., Pittet, V., Rossel, J. B., von Känel, R., Anderegg, C., Bauerfeind, P., ... & Thorens, J. (2016). Symptoms of depression and anxiety are independently associated with clinical recurrence of inflammatory bowel disease. *Clinical Gastroenterology and Hepatology, 14*(6), 829–835.

Moulton, C. D., Pavlidis, P., Norton, C., Norton, S., Pariante, C., Hayee, B. & Powell, N. (2019). Depressive symptoms in inflammatory bowel disease: an extraintestinal manifestation of inflammation? *Clinical & Experimental Immunology, 197*(3), 308–318.

Neuendorf, R., Harding, A., Stello, N., Hanes, D. & Wahbeh, H. (2016). Depression and anxiety in patients with inflammatory bowel disease: a systematic review. *Journal of Psychosomatic Research, 87*, 70–80.

Nowakowski, J., Chrobak, A. A. & Dudek, D. (2016). Psychiatric illnesses in inflammatory bowel diseases — psychiatric comorbidity and biological underpinnings. *Psychiatria Polska, 50*(6), 1157–1166.

Pérez-Vigil, A., de la Cruz, L. F., Brander, G., Isomura, K., Gromark, C. & Mataix-Cols, D. (2016). The link between autoimmune diseases and obsessive-compulsive and tic disorders: a systematic review. *Neuroscience & Biobehavioral Reviews, 71*, 542–562.

Reinhorn, I. M., Bernstein, C. N., Graff, L. A., Patten, S. B., Sareen, J., Fisk, J. D., Bolton, J. M., Hitchon, C. & Marrie, R. A. (2020). Social phobia in immune-mediated inflammatory diseases. *Journal of Psychosomatic Research, 128*, 109890.

Robelin, K., Senada, P., Ghoz, H., Sim, L., Lebow, J., Picco, M., Cangemi, J., Farraye, F. A. & Werlang, M. (2021). Prevalence and clinician recognition of avoidant/restrictive food intake disorder in patients with inflammatory bowel disease. *Gastroenterology & Hepatology, 17*(11), 510.

Taft, T. H., Ballou, S., Bedell, A. & Lincenberg, D. (2017). Psychological considerations and interventions in inflammatory bowel disease patient care. *Gastroenterology Clinics, 46*(4), 847–858.

Taft, T. H., Bedell, A., Craven, M. R., Guadagnoli, L., Quinton, S. & Hanauer, S. B. (2019). Initial assessment of post-traumatic stress in a US cohort of inflammatory bowel disease patients. *Inflammatory Bowel Diseases, 25*(9), 1577–1585.

Taft, T. H. & Keefer, L. (2016). A systematic review of disease-related stigmatization in patients living with inflammatory bowel disease. *Clinical and Experimental Gastroenterology*, 49–58.

Yelencich, E., Truong, E., Widaman, A. M., Pignotti, G., Yang, L., Jeon, Y., Weber, A., T., Shah, R., Smith, J., Sauk, J. S. & Limketkai, B. N. (2022). Avoidant restrictive food intake disorder prevalent among patients with inflammatory bowel disease. *Clinical Gastroenterology and Hepatology, 20*(6), 1282–1289.

Eight Session CBT Protocol for IBD **5**

What follows in this chapter is a set of loose guidelines for a session by session protocol intended to last about eight sessions. Please note that unlike many manualized, empirically supported treatments, the eight session format will be too many sessions for some patients, and not nearly enough for others. In Part III, which provides a number of hypothetical patient protocols, you will see that some patients truly only need four to five sessions, while others may need psychosocial therapeutic support for years. However, many patients can be helped a great deal in about eight sessions.

The following modules will point the clinician toward flexible deployment of numerous empirically supported principles and transdiagnostic techniques and interventions, with a good understanding of how the IBD may be central to the person's distress. We will start with the first two sessions, which will be quite similar for most patients. We will then move on to modules that can be mixed and matched, depending on what the patient is struggling with.

Session 1

Start by setting an agenda. "This session is mostly a chance for me to get to know you. I want to hear your story. I'll probably ask a few clarifying questions along the way, but this will be your chance to share your history with me—a little about your life, where you grew up, your family, education, and work history, but also the history of your experience with your IBD. Then I want to be sure to save about ten minutes at the end to teach you a very specific skill

DOI: 10.4324/9781003454380-8

called deep diaphragmatic breathing. So really the ball's in your court. Let me know if there is anything else you think it's important for us to cover."

As with any new patient, the therapist's first job is to take a thorough history. This will include a standard psychosocial assessment, but will have a special focus on the patient's IBD, including their current physical health and medications. Many patients can fill an entire hour sharing the "saga" of the development of their illness, their diagnostic journey, any treatment they've undergone, and their current health status. For many patients, it can be therapeutic to simply tell their story to a knowledgeable listener who is willing to take the time to hear them out, who understands and can anticipate the challenges, and who will not recoil or be disgusted by the details.

You should be sure to come to a clear understanding of the current status of their illness (Are they in remission? Are they maintained on medication? Are they still symptomatic, either due to ongoing inflammation or secondary IBS?). You should try to get a sense of the degree to which their IBD interferes with their life or causes disability or distress, either because of active symptoms, because of dietary restrictions or because of maladaptive coping strategies such as secrecy and avoidance.

Session 1 should *always* end with ten minutes to teach deep diaphragmatic breathing (DDB). Explain to the patient that deep breathing, when done correctly, recruits parasympathetic nervous system activation (rest and *digest*) throughout the entire body. It reduces the impact of stress on every body system, AND it optimizes intestinal motility. Particularly for people with secondary IBS, this can be enormously helpful. Some CBT therapists learned at some point in their training *not* to teach DDB, because it could, in principle, be used as an avoidance strategy or a safety utilization behavior in people experiencing panic, social anxiety, and PTSD or could even become a compulsion in OCD. Sometimes DDB is even compared to Xanax or other benzodiazepines, and is assumed to interfere with the efficacy of exposure therapy. Please put aside those beliefs right now. There is good data (e.g., from Alicia Meuret's work) that respiratory retraining leads to reductions in panic symptom severity mediated by changes in appraisal and increased perceived control. Even in OCD, DDB can facilitate exposure therapy by making approach behaviors easier to tolerate and therefore more likely to be engaged in. Whatever your beliefs about the value of DDB in patients with primary anxiety disorders, it is incredibly important to teach it effectively to GI patients. Anxiety and sympathetic arousal have a direct biological effect on activity in the gut, exacerbating discomfort, tightness, cramping, urgency, and even the possibility of fecal incontinence.

By teaching patients to reduce sympathetic arousal and increase parasympathetic arousal, you give them a crucial tool in managing their GI symptoms. This isn't just about *perceived* control. It is about *actual* control. Many patients with IBD feel betrayed by their bodies. Some even feel like their body has become an alien enemy that can turn on them at any moment. They can't trust their body to maintain basic functions like digestion and continence. Anxiety about urgency and fecal incontinence aren't catastrophic distortions. They are very real possibilities. DDB is one of the most effective tools we have available to us to calm down a crampy gut and buy time to get to a bathroom. This is even more true for patients who have developed secondary IBS. For many IBS patients, DDB can actually stop the cramping completely, leading to a dramatic reduction in anxiety and life interference.

Here is a basic script you can use to teach DDB effectively. "Now I'm going to teach you to do something called deep diaphragmatic breathing. Deep breathing is a super helpful way to reduce stress and can even help reduce GI symptoms like cramping and urgency. You've heard of "fight or flight" right? That's sympathetic nervous system arousal, and it's what our body does when we are stressed or anxious or rising to a challenge. Fewer people have heard what the parasympathetic nervous system does—it's responsible for "rest" and my favorite, "digest." The parasympathetic system is active when all is right with the world and we can relax and digest our food. Together, the sympathetic and parasympathetic systems make up the autonomic, or "automatic" nervous system. That means that all those processes happen automatically. We don't have to think about them. That's a good thing! If we had to remember to keep our heart beating, and we got distracted, we'd die! So we can't really directly control most of the parts of this system. If I asked you to "lower your blood pressure" right now, or to "tell your liver to start storing extra glucose as glycogen" you wouldn't know what muscle to squeeze. But the good news is that there is ONE part of this system over which we can *choose* to exert conscious control when we want to. And that is … the breath. And the really good news is that the breath is wired into every other part of the autonomic nervous system. So by changing how we breathe, we can either activate the sympathetic nervous system or the parasympathetic nervous system."

"Now most people have heard the advice to "just take a deep breath" when you're feeling stressed or angry. And for most people, it doesn't really help. It turns out that's because most people are doing it wrong. So let me see you take a deep breath right now."

Watch carefully while the patient takes a "deep" breath. The vast majority of people will actually take a shallow thoracic breath. Their upper chest will rise, their shoulders will move toward their ears, and the tendons in their neck may even stand out. If this happens, say:

"Wonderful! That was terrible. It's wonderful because it means I have something to teach you that is going to be a real game changer. You just did what 99% of people do when told to take a deep breath. It's what you do in the doctor's office when the doctor puts the stethoscope on your chest and says 'take a deep breath.' This is what you just did—watch me." Now replicate the shallow thoracic breath with the rising chest, shoulders, and tight neck. Suggest that they watch you as you do it again and focus on your neck muscles and tendons. Ask them "does that look relaxing?" Most patients will immediately say no. Say "That's exactly right. That's not a relaxing breath at all. Now I'm going to teach you how to do it in a way that will feel totally different. Let's both stand up. (If delivering therapy remotely via video, ask the person to stand up, step back from the camera, and angle the device so that you can see them from the hips to the face.) Now the first thing we're going to do is just find the muscle we're going to use. Don't worry about breathing just yet." Turn slightly sideways so the patient can see your abdomen and chest in a partial profile. "Put one hand on your abdomen just below your belly button, and pretend you're in a swimsuit commercial. Just suck in your gut, and then let it out." Keep doing this with the patient four to five times. Then say "You should start to feel some muscle burn right under your rib cage. Got it? That's your diaphragm!

"Now the next thing we're going to do is exhale." Pick up a tissue so you can demonstrate this. Hold one hand up in front of you holding the tissue and keep the other hand on your belly. "I'm going to pretend I'm blowing out a candle. You'll see the tissue flutter as my exhale blows on it. I'm going to squeeze the diaphragm muscle, just like we were just doing, but this time I'm going to use that to force the air out of my lungs. Just like squeezing a balloon will force the air out, I'm going to squeeze my belly muscles to force the air out of my lungs." Demonstrate this two to three times, being sure they can see your belly contracting and the tissue fluttering. "Now you try it. Just pretend you're blowing out a candle." Praise the patient for doing this and say "Great. Now the next thing we're going to do is blow out all the candles on my last birthday cake (or some similar joke). That's a LOT of candles! To blow out that many candles, we need a long, slow sustained exhale. I'm going to exhale for a full eight seconds now. When I'm done exhaling, I'm just going to relax my belly muscles and let them soften, and the air will pour back into my lungs. Watch me first." Now demo this with a long slow exhale through pursed lips. You can show the count of the seconds passing by holding up a finger with each second. "Now you try it." Observe the patient closely as they do it, counting out loud. Have them exhale first, and then coach them through the inhale by saying "Now relax, soften and let the air pour back in-five-six-hold!   Exhale-two-three-four-five-six-seven-eight-Inhale-soften-three-four-five-six-hold! Exhale-two … etc." Go through four breaths this way. Then stop and ask the patient how that feels. Most people will say something like "Wow—weirdly relaxing." Say "Right!? Now go back and take one of those shallow thoracic breaths you took at the beginning." Wait for them to do it, and then ask "How does that feel in comparison?" Again, most patients will notice right away that the shallow breath actually makes them feel more tense and keyed up, while the true deep breath makes them feel more relaxed. If the patient reports instead that the DDB is making them feel lightheaded, have them practice again but hold their breath at the top of the inhale for a few seconds. Continue to practice until they report that it does indeed feel relaxing. Then drive the message home. "This is a fantastic bio-hack for turning on the parasympathetic nervous system and helping your body rest and digest. Deep breathing actually optimizes intestinal motility, and it can help reduce cramping and urgency and give you time to get to a bathroom. In other words, it gives us a measure of control over body processes that are normally totally outside of conscious control."

For patients who are particularly sophisticated and/or curious about underlying biological processes, you can explain the concepts of heart rate variability (HRV) and respiratory sinus arrhythmia (RSA). RSA happens naturally during the breath cycle. During the inhale, heart rate typically speeds up a bit. During the exhale, a branch of the vaso-vagal nerve (the main nerve of the parasympathetic system) engages on the heart and slows it down, acting like a kind of brake. This means that over the course of a breath (respiratory) the sinus rhythm of the heart changes (hence arrhythmia). We normally think of the word arrhythmia as a bad thing, but in this case it is part of the normal electrophysiology of the heart. DDB exaggerates RSA, but also leads to lower heart rate overall. Heart rate variability is measured in a number of different ways, but the easiest to understand is the SDNN, or the standard deviation (SD) of the normal to normal (NN) beats of the heart. That is, how variable is your pulse over time. Somewhat counter-intuitively, higher HRV (that is a more variable heart rate) is actually a sign of both good cardiovascular health *and* effective emotion regulation. Again, slow DDB elevates HRV over time, precisely because it is exaggerating RSA.

The homework assigned for Week 1 follows naturally from this exercise.

Homework for Week 1: Practice deep diaphragmatic breathing three times a day for one minute at a time. Shoot for a respiration rate of four breaths per minute, with an eight second exhale, six second inhale, and holding the breath for two seconds. Point out that while that might seem very slow (normal ambulatory respiration is around 16–20 breaths per minute), it is actually what you were just doing with them! After a few days, see if they can use DDB to reduce cramping and urgency. If their IBD is well controlled medically, they may well be able to reduce urgency and discomfort by doing this. (If they are still suffering from active inflammation, DDB may not help much at all with burning pain and urgency, but can still help people relax and cope with other stressors in their lives.) Even if it doesn't help with GI symptoms, DDB is a wonderful way to de-stress and is the single most useful relaxation strategy for folks with GI disorders.

One fun way to combine cheap, on the fly biofeedback training with DDB, is to have the patient use a fitness watch or inexpensive pulse oximeter (available at any pharmacy or from Amazon) to watch their heart rate in real time while they practice DDB.[1] They should notice that their heart rate accelerates during and at the very end of the inhale, and then slows down during the exhale. Over a minute or two, they should also notice that their overall heart rate declines. I like to show people that I can move my pulse around by 20 beats per minute just by changing how I breathe. I can shoot it up to around 85 by taking lots of quick, shallow chest breaths, and then I can lower it down to about 65 by taking four to five deep diaphragmatic breaths. It's a pretty compelling demonstration, especially if they can achieve the same thing in session with you, or during their homework practice. This is especially helpful for patients who are skeptical that "talk therapy" can bring about any changes in underlying biological processes, much less autoimmune related diseases.

---

[1] This is another place where DEI and health disparities may need to be taken into account. Most of these devices depend on the LED light reflected off the skin back to the sensor. The measurement of both heart rate and oxygen saturation may well be inaccurate when the devices are used by dark-skinned people, since melanin alters the skin's light absorption and reflection.

It's a very concrete example of how a learned skill can bring about a concrete change in a biological process they thought they had no control over.

Session 2

As in any CBT protocol, Session 2 should begin with a review of the homework. Ask the patient how the DDB went. Watch them take a few deep breaths and ensure that they are doing it correctly. Some patients need extra practice to shift their breath to true DDB, rather than shallow thoracic breaths. Encourage them to practice lying down if they are struggling with this skill. If the patient still has active GI symptoms, ask about whether they tried it when they were feeling cramping and urgency. Many patients will report that it did seem to "take the edge off" abdominal pain and urgency and gave them a little window in which to get to the bathroom.

After the homework review, finish taking their history and begin to establish which, if any, psychological diagnosis (or diagnoses) they might meet criteria for. This is a good time to ask about dietary restrictions and the possibility of an ARFID diagnosis, any catastrophic fears they might have (e.g., fecal incontinence or needing an ostomy) and any avoidance behaviors they are engaging in. The goal of Session 2 is to build a case conceptualization and to identify collaboratively with the patient what the most important targets are for treatment.

The homework for Session 2 will depend entirely on the case conceptualization and the patient's goals for treatment. For example, if the patient experiences a great deal of shame about their disease, and keeps it secret even from close friends and loved ones, a good assignment is to have them identify one individual they trust who doesn't know about their illness, and then have them *tell* that individual that they have a chronic GI disorder. You can practice with the patient how they might go about raising it and talking about it. Say something like "I just want you to know that I have a chronic medical condition that affects my digestive system. I mostly manage it pretty well, but sometimes I need to restrict what I eat, and sometimes I need to use the bathroom more frequently. I take medicine for it that works pretty well, but does make me vulnerable to other infections, like sinus infections. That's why I may need to excuse myself sometimes, or bring my own food to gatherings, or take time off to recover from upper respiratory infections." Often when they hear the therapist model such a disclosure in a matter of fact way they will say "Well it doesn't sound so terrible when *you* say it."

On the other hand, if the patient is deathly afraid that a wide variety of foods will set off their symptoms, but has been encouraged by a registered dietician to expand their diet, you can set a very modest exposure assignment for this week. Encourage them to try a few bites of a single feared food (e.g., yogurt or oatmeal) several days in a row to see what happens. This assumes that you have a good understanding of any actual medical restrictions they are working with. Some patients are very committed to following the Specific Carbohydrate Diet, the IBD Anti-Inflammatory Diet (IBD-AID), or the Low FODMAP Diet. It is notable that both the IBD-AID and the Low FODMAP Diet are supposed to unfold in stages, with the maintenance phase being the least restrictive phase possible.

If the patient's primary difficulty is agoraphobia secondary to fear of fecal incontinence, then a good homework assignment might be to have them visit a few shops and ask to use the restroom as a medical emergency, on a day when they are actually feeling fine, so the assignment has relatively low stakes.

The point is that treatment from here on out will be specific to each individual patient, but will rely on a number of basic transdiagnostic principles and techniques (e.g., cognitive reappraisal and de-catastrophizing, behavioral experiments, exposure therapy to overcome maladaptive avoidance, and so on). What follows is a sample session format, but therapists should feel free to mix and match when they introduce interventions like thought records or exposure.

Session 3

Introduce the cognitive model of stress management. Identify one or two cognitive distortions or catastrophic fears or beliefs the person holds. Be sure to inquire about fear of fecal incontinence, shame, and secrecy. This is the time to break out thought records and explain the basic model of how our thoughts about situations determine how we feel about them. Most experienced CBT therapists have their own way of introducing this, whether they frame it as the ABC model (activating event, belief, consequence) or whether they use the same hypothetical example with every patient. ("Imagine you see an acquaintance walking down the other side of the street in the opposite direction and you wave and the person doesn't wave back. How would you feel? What thought is that based on? What if the person just didn't see you?") Pull out a few blank thought records and have the patient complete them in session with you. For their homework, send them home with a few blank thought records and ask them to complete them over the course of the week. They might use events in which their GI symptoms were flaring, or they were having distressing thoughts about IBD related experiences or symptoms, or they might just choose events that have nothing to do with their IBD. The goal is to teach them this tried and true approach to reducing unnecessary stress in their lives. Figure 5.1 is a blank thought record of the kind I use, along with an example that has been completed in session with a patient (Figure 5.2).

Session 4

Introduce exposure therapy and behavioral experiments. Examples include walking into random stores and asking to use the bathroom, telling a friend or colleague about the IBD, reintroducing a (medically approved) but feared food into their diet, going out to a restaurant, etc. If the patient is resistant to trying exposure therapy, this might be a good time to introduce a decisional balancing exercise from motivational interviewing. Have them identify a behavior they are ambivalent about changing. This could be driving, eating a feared food, talking to a loved one about their IBD, or going for a walk—any target of change that seems like it would actually improve their HRQL and reduce disability long term that they are afraid of or resistant to trying. Then have them complete a two by two grid identifying the pros and cons of both trying to change the behavior and not trying to change the behavior. This is a novel exercise for most people, since we often only consider the pros and cons of *doing* something, not the pros and cons of *not* doing something. Encourage people to fill the boxes out honestly—what they *actually* believe, not what they think they "should" put in the box. I like to get people to "rate" the boxes on a scale of 1 to 10, where the rating is some combination of how important or compelling the box feels, and how much they believe it. An example of an initial completed decisional balancing exercise is shown in Figure 5.3.

A quick glance at the numbers reveals that the person's motivation to do the exposure exercise and try walking her son to his daycare is less than her motivation to avoid doing it. Motivation is always the sum total of the

Objective Situation	Thoughts and Beliefs	Outcome Feelings and Behavior	Rational Response

Figure 5.1 Blank thought record

Objective Situation	Thoughts and Beliefs	Outcome Feelings and Behavior	Rational Response
A new friend has invited me to go to a show with them.	I can't do this. What if I'm at the concert and I have to go to the bathroom urgently? I'll have to leave the hall, climbing over people, and I'll miss the act. My friend will be super annoyed that they wasted the ticket on me. It will be embarrassing and will inconvenience everyone. Even if I can manage to wait until intermission, if there's a line I might not make it in time. And if there are a lot of people waiting it will be rude to occupy a stall and stink the place up. I should just say no. This sucks because they may think I don't like them.	Super anxious. Embarrassed. Sad. Lonely.	The new medication is working pretty well and I haven't had that much urgency lately. My doctor said it's okay to take some Imodium when I need to. If I eat a light lunch and take two to three Imodium I should be fine. Even if I do have to go to the bathroom, it would be inconvenient and annoying but it doesn't have to ruin the evening. People are actually pretty understanding if you say you truly have an emergency and need to go right away. If I explain to my friend that I really want to go, and let them know that I may have issues, hopefully they'll be understanding. Saying no to things like this is what makes me feel isolated and lonely and sad. Even if the evening doesn't go exactly as I hope, it's still worth the risk.

Figure 5.2 Example completed thought record

Decision	Pros	Cons
Continue letting my husband drop our son off at daycare.	Easier for me. Way less stress. I won't have to worry about taking Imodium and half a Xanax every morning. I can relax at home and then start my (remote) work day. 6	My husband is really busy with work. He's getting frustrated and annoyed with me. I'm missing time with our son. It's embarrassing that I can't do this. I feel pathetic. 6
Drop my son off at daycare myself.	My husband will be relieved and less annoyed with me. I'm his mother—I should be able to do this. I would feel brave and normal if I could actually do it (but I don't think I can). Maybe I could make a few new friends (but that feels unlikely). 5	Scary! I might experience urgency. What if I can't get to the bathroom in time? I might have a panic attack. I'll have to "chat" with other parents while we wait to sign in. I'll feel trapped. Other parents will notice my discomfort and anxiety. I'll be humiliated. I'll have to load up on Imodium and Xanax just to face it. 10

Figure 5.3 Example of a completed decisional balancing worksheet

perceived benefits of doing the thing plus the perceived costs of not doing the thing, weighed against the perceived benefits of not doing the thing and the perceived costs of doing it. In other words, her motivation to try to walk her son to daycare is the sum of the cost of letting her husband keep doing it (6) plus the possible benefits of doing it herself (5) which adds up to 11. But her motivation to keep avoiding it is the sum of the benefits of letting her

Decision	Pros	Cons
Continue letting my husband drop our son off at daycare.	Easier for me. Less stressful, *but I might be making more of this than I should.* I won't have to worry about taking Imodium and half a Xanax every morning. I can relax at home and then start my (remote) work day. 5	My husband is really busy with work. *I should take this off his plate.* He's getting frustrated and annoyed with me. *I hate how much conflict it causes.* I'm missing time with our son *which makes me really sad.* *I don't want my son to think I'm incapable.* It's embarrassing that I can't do this. I feel pathetic. 8
Drop my son off at daycare myself.	My husband will be relieved *and things might get much better between us. It would be really nice to have less conflict with him.* *It could be a sweet bonding time with my son.* I'm his mother—I should be able to do this. I'll feel *brave for trying* and *eventually it might even feel normal.* Maybe I can make a few new friends—*that one mom seemed friendly last time I was there.* 7	Scary urgency? *I've been practicing the deep breathing and I've never actually experienced incontinence.* *There is a coffee shop on the way to daycare. If I need to stop I can.* I might have a panic attack *but I know that's just uncomfortable, not dangerous.* I'll have to "chat" with other parents while we wait to sign in—*true but that's how you make friends.* Other parents might notice my discomfort and anxiety, *but probably not, and even if they do, so what?*

Figure 5.4 Revised decisional balancing worksheet

Decision	Pros	Cons
		I'll have to take Imodium and Xanax to manage it at first. *My doctor says Imodium is fine, so I shouldn't worry about that. With practice I may be able to wean off the Xanax.*
		5

Figure 5.4 *(continued)*

husband do it (6) plus the potential costs of trying to do it herself (10) which adds up to 16. The numbers don't lie. As much as she may "want" to be able to walk her son to daycare, if she keeps thinking about it this way she'll never overcome the motivational deficit. Figure 5.4 shows a revised decisional balancing worksheet after she and the therapist discuss the various pros and cons and do some cognitive reappraisal.

She was able to identify that it makes her really *sad* to not walk her son to daycare. Being an engaged and loving mother is a core value for her, and her sadness over that is more motivating than dealing with her husband's irritation. She also upped her confidence that some of the good things might actually be possible, like having a better relationship with her husband and bonding time with her son. Most of the movement, however, was in reducing the cons of walking her son. She was doing a lot of catastrophizing in her initial analysis. By reducing the perceived costs of trying to make the change, she shifted the motivational balance enough. Now her motivation to try walking her son is 8 plus 7 which equals 15. Her motivation to avoid walking her son is now 5 plus 5, or 10. The balance has changed enough and she might well be willing to give it a try.

Of course, when you are designing exposure therapy assignments, you want to set the patient up for success. There is considerable debate in the field at the moment as to the best way to structure exposure therapy. There is certainly evidence from both animal and human studies that inhibitory learning can be enhanced by various strategies including expectancy violation, removal of safety signals, attentional focus, deepened extinction, stimulus variability, occasional reinforced extinction, and enhancing retrieval of inhibitory learning via multiple contexts and retrieval cues. While I understand

and admire the translational science behind these modifications, I personally prefer to use old fashioned graded exposure and within session habituation. It is a gentler approach that is easier for patients to tolerate and buy into, especially if they fear fecal incontinence.

Session 5

If there is any trauma history related to the IBD, this might be a good time to initiate trauma focused treatment. Encourage the person to share the story. Empathize, validate, and reframe if possible. Examples include episodes of actual incontinence (or close calls), emergency room visits, hospitalizations or surgeries, interactions with incompetent or invalidating physicians, and teasing or shaming by others. Now is a good time to cover anger at any mismanagement of the disease they have experienced, and to encourage collaborative, proactive care with their current physician. As covered in Chapter 4, you may or may not need to use techniques or full protocols from Prolonged Exposure, Cognitive Processing Therapy, Eye Movement Desensitization and Reprocessing or Imaginal Rescripting (the main empirically supported trauma treatments), but you should certainly have the patient revisit that difficult history, even if they don't meet criteria for PTSD. If there is no trauma history, use this session to continue exploring exposure therapy and cognitive reappraisal.

Session 6

Encourage continued exposure therapy and cognitive reappraisal. If there is resistance to using medication as prescribed or recommended, explore beliefs and concerns. For example, if their physician has said it is fine to use Imodium or a bile acid sequestrant to manage diarrhea, but the person resists doing it for fear of developing an obstruction, encourage them to consider overall quality of life and to discuss the likelihood of the feared outcome with their doctor. If their doctor has recommended surgery or a new biologic drug or a round of steroids, but they are very reluctant to pursue it, help them think it through, including in their analysis the risks of NOT undergoing surgery, or taking the medication.

For some patients, this might be a good time to suggest a medication consult for a neuromodulator that can serve as an antidepressant or anti-anxiety medication. Good candidates include medications from the SNRI group (including duloxetine, venlafaxine, and desvenlafaxine) or the old tricyclic antidepressants (including imipramine, amitriptyline, and nortriptyline). At the right dose, all of these medications can reduce urgency and diarrhea, and may address abdominal pain as well. Of course, they can also worsen constipation, which can be problematic for *some* patients with IBD, though not all. SSRIs (such as fluoxetine, sertraline, or citalopram) are often not appropriate, since they tend to make diarrhea worse, but this is highly variable from patient to patient. If you can find a good psychiatrist with some knowledge of integrated health and GI, they can generally make highly informed and useful recommendations to your patient. Many gastroenterologists are also comfortable prescribing these medications as adjunctive care for IBD.

Session 7

Use this session flexibly to address ongoing disease management, self-care and relaxation strategies. This can be a good time to incorporate mindfulness and acceptance skills. I like to teach a sequence of attention training exercises. The first one covers mindful awareness of sounds and skin temperature, then a full body scan (excluding visceral or abdominal sensations), breath awareness, and then heartbeat. Mindfulness is a very useful skill for people with chronic health conditions, especially those that involve pain. Ultimately the goal is to get people to learn to disengage their attention and emotional investment from uncomfortable physical sensations and thoughts. You can end the session with this exercise, with homework being to practice mindfulness (using Headspace, Calm, Mindfulness Coach, or free videos on YouTube) over the course of the week. In addition to its track record in helping with chronic pain, incorporating mindfulness based interventions (MBIs) into CBT has been shown to reduce relapse in a number of disorders. If you are unfamiliar with MBIs, I strongly encourage you to seek continuing education and to consider experimenting with practicing mindfulness yourself. While you do not need to attend a full blown certification program in Mindfulness Based Stress Reduction (MBSR) in order to extend some of the benefits of mindfulness to your patients, I do suggest some specific training and a nascent mindfulness practice yourself. It will help you guide and direct patients appropriately.

Session 8

Sense of self and IBD, review and termination. Encourage your patient to see themselves as an active manager of their disease, but not as defined by the disease. Review their progress and any improvement they have made in identifying and addressing catastrophic beliefs and in reducing avoidance behavior. You can do a second mindful attention training exercise in this session. This time, incorporate awareness of visceral sensations and discomfort, but have the person shift their attention back and forth between the breath and abdominal sensations several times. Guide them to hold open, curious awareness of abdominal sensations and then shift their attention *away* from them. They will not learn this skill in just a few sessions, but by giving them a template for what they are trying to accomplish, they can continue to practice on their own with the guidance of a good app.

For many patients, especially those who started with only mild or recent onset psychiatric comorbidity, an eight session protocol similar to this one will be sufficient. Indeed, for some, it will be too many sessions. But for others, especially those with more severe psychopathology, longer standing problems, or more severe or poorly controlled IBD, eight sessions may not be nearly enough. Some folks will benefit from further treatment that may have little to do with their IBD. Perhaps they are stuck in their careers, want to work on their relationship, or need help with parenting a difficult teenager. They may have long standing depression or social anxiety, or OCD that actually predated the IBD and they could still benefit from therapy. Some folks just need *support*. IBD can be tough to live with. Even if they have learned new skills, addressed catastrophizing, and reduced avoidance, they may want to continue to have a safe space with a knowledgeable and empathetic therapist who can continue to provide guidance, advocacy and emotional support.

If the patient is ready to terminate therapy, celebrate! It can be very important to remind people of where they were when they started, and how far they have come. Sometimes patients think that the improvements they have experienced in mood and quality of life are somehow magical, or due entirely to the mysterious machinations of the therapist. Always remind patients of the hard work they themselves did and the skills they learned. This is important, because it reminds them that they will be able to continue using those skills moving forward.

I usually assure my patients that I'm not going anywhere. If they need a session in a few months they can always call. Because I am in a private practice model, and have total control of my own schedule, it is easy for me to fit people in for a few booster sessions on an ad hoc basis. Therapists working in hospitals, or large group practice settings may have less control over their schedules. But if possible, it's a good idea to let people know that if things get difficult for them, you're happy to step back in. Most folks won't need to take advantage of this, but it can be a relief to them to know you're available.

Termination sessions are often delightful. It gives both the patient and the therapist a chance to reflect on the shared work and the progress the patient made and how much better their life is overall. Even if their IBD is still problematic, most patients agree that their quality of life has gotten much better. It can be deeply satisfying work for all concerned.

Summary

This chapter outlined a basic overview of an eight session treatment protocol using a variety of CBT based strategies for addressing the common problems that patients with IBD might present with. Some of the sessions included specific scripts (like the DDB training script for the first session) or examples of specific exercises (like thoughts records in Session 3 and a motivational interviewing decisional balancing worksheet for increasing motivation to engage in exposure therapy in Session 4). Most of the sessions, however, outline general goals and transdiagnostic techniques that *might* make sense to introduce in a particular week, but might be better placed at some other time, or might not be necessary at all (for example, trauma focused work if the patient does not actually report any history of trauma). Of necessity, this protocol is somewhat modular, and the suggested format and schedule is just that—a suggestion. It will be up to the individual therapist to use their wisdom, experience, clinical acumen, and skills to address the issues raised by each individual patient. The good news is that all of your standard CBT skills will work well with this patient population, as long as you bring extra knowledge about the ins and outs of IBD with you to the work.

Bibliography

Bennebroek Evertsz, F., Sprangers, M. A., Sitnikova, K., Stokkers, P. C., Ponsioen, C. Y., Bartelsman, J. F., ... & Bockting, C. L. (2017). Effectiveness of cognitive–behavioral therapy on quality of life, anxiety, and depressive symptoms among patients with inflammatory bowel disease: A multicenter randomized controlled trial. *Journal of Consulting and Clinical Psychology, 85*(9), 918.

Bonaz, B., Sinniger, V. & Pellissier, S. (2016). Vagal tone: effects on sensitivity, motility, and inflammation. *Neurogastroenterology & Motility, 28*(4), 455–462.

Bosch, M. & Arntz, A. (2023). Imagery rescripting for patients with posttraumatic stress disorder: a qualitative study of patients' and therapists' perspectives about the elements of change. *Cognitive and Behavioral Practice, 30*(1), 18–34.

Craven, M. R., Quinton, S. & Taft, T. H. (2019). Inflammatory bowel disease patient experiences with psychotherapy in the community. *Journal of Clinical Psychology in Medical Settings, 26*, 183–193.

Ewais, T., Begun, J., Kenny, M., Rickett, K., Hay, K., Ajilchi, B. & Kisely, S. (2019). A systematic review and meta-analysis of mindfulness based interventions and yoga in inflammatory bowel disease. *Journal of Psychosomatic Research, 116*, 44–53.

Feingold, J., Murray, H. B. & Keefer, L. (2019). Recent advances in cognitive behavioral therapy for digestive disorders and the role of applied positive psychology across the spectrum of GI care. *Journal of Clinical Gastroenterology, 53*(7), 477–485.

Gholamrezaei, A., Van Diest, I., Aziz, Q., Pauwels, A., Tack, J., Vlaeyen, J. W. & Van Oudenhove, L. (2022). Effect of slow, deep breathing on visceral pain perception and its underlying psychophysiological mechanisms. *Neurogastroenterology & Motility, 34*(4), e14242.

Hamasaki, H. (2020). Effects of diaphragmatic breathing on health: a narrative review. *Medicines, 7*(10), 65.

Hardcastle, S. J., Fortier, M., Blake, N. & Hagger, M. S. (2017). Identifying content-based and relational techniques to change behaviour in motivational interviewing. *Health Psychology Review, 11*(1), 1–16.

Hood, M. M. & Jedel, S. (2017). Mindfulness-based interventions in inflammatory bowel disease. *Gastroenterology Clinics, 46*(4), 859–874.

Hopper, S. I., Murray, S. L., Ferrara, L. R. & Singleton, J. K. (2019). Effectiveness of diaphragmatic breathing for reducing physiological and psychological stress in adults: a quantitative systematic review. *JBI Evidence Synthesis, 17*(9), 1855–1876.

Hunt, M. G. (2021). *Coping with Crohn's and Colitis: A Patient and Clinician's Guide to CBT for IBD*. Routledge.

Hunt, M. G., Rushton, J., Shenberger, E. & Murayama, S. (2018). Positive effects of diaphragmatic breathing on physiological stress reactivity in varsity athletes. *Journal of Clinical Sport Psychology, 12*(1), 27–38.

Keefer, L., Bedell, A., Norton, C. & Hart, A. L. (2022). How should pain, fatigue, and emotional wellness be incorporated into treatment goals for optimal management of inflammatory bowel disease? *Gastroenterology, 162*(5), 1439–1451.

King, L. A., Urbach, J. R. & Stewart, K. E. (2015). Illness anxiety and avoidant/restrictive food intake disorder: cognitive-behavioral conceptualization and treatment. *Eating Behaviors, 19*, 106–109.

Laborde, S., Allen, M. S., Borges, U., Dosseville, F., Hosang, T. J., Iskra, M., Mosley, E., Salvotti, C., Spolverato, L., Zammit, N. & Javelle, F. (2022). Effects of voluntary slow breathing on heart rate and heart rate variability: a systematic review and a meta-analysis. *Neuroscience & Biobehavioral Reviews, 138*, 104711.

McClintock, A. S., McCarrick, S. M., Garland, E. L., Zeidan, F. & Zgierska, A. E. (2019). Brief mindfulness-based interventions for acute and chronic pain: a systematic review. *The Journal of Alternative and Complementary Medicine, 25*(3), 265–278.

Meuret, A. E. & Ritz, T. (2021). Capnometry-assisted respiratory training. *Principles and Practice of Stress Management, 303.*

Mikocka-Walus, A., Andrews, J. M. & Bampton, P. (2016). Cognitive behavioral therapy for IBD. *Inflammatory Bowel Diseases, 22*(2), E5–E6.

Miller, W. R. & Rose, G. S. (2015). Motivational interviewing and decisional balance: contrasting responses to client ambivalence. *Behavioural and Cognitive Psychotherapy, 43*(2), 129–141.

Naude, C., Skvarc, D., Knowles, S., Russell, L., Evans, S. & Mikocka-Walus, A. (2023). The effectiveness of mindfulness-based interventions in inflammatory bowel disease: a systematic review & meta-analysis. *Journal of Psychosomatic Research, 111232.*

Raabe, S., Ehring, T., Marquenie, L., Arntz, A. & Kindt, M. (2022). Imagery rescripting as a stand-alone treatment for posttraumatic stress disorder related to childhood abuse: a randomized controlled trial. *Journal of Behavior Therapy and Experimental Psychiatry, 77*, 101769.

Salwen-Deremer, J. K., Siegel, C. A. & Smith, M. T. (2020). Cognitive behavioral therapy for insomnia: a promising treatment for insomnia, pain, and depression in patients with IBD. *Crohn's & Colitis 360, 2*(3).

Spoelstra, S. L., Schueller, M., Hilton, M. & Ridenour, K. (2015). Interventions combining motivational interviewing and cognitive behaviour to promote medication adherence: a literature review. *Journal of Clinical Nursing, 24*(9–10), 1163–1173.

Part III

Therapy in Action

Sample Treatment Protocols

6

Introduction to Treatment Protocols

These treatment protocols are illustrative examples of various kinds of patients with IBD. While the cases differ considerably in many details (age and sex of patient, severity and type of IBD, psychiatric comorbidity, and so on) there are also parallels between them all, and the treatment protocols follow a recognizable arc. Assuming you are experienced with CBT more generally, reading through these treatment protocols should give you a good idea of how to apply CBT specifically to patients with an IBD. If you are somewhat less familiar with CBT principles and approaches, I hope these case summaries will help you appreciate the power and the flexibility and scope of the approach. CBT is often caricatured as a collection of "techniques," that ignores the therapeutic relationship, and doesn't pay attention to the patient's history or their current context and family system. Nothing could be further from the truth. CBT is a comprehensive system of psychotherapy that takes into account early development, family history, and current context and functioning. Moreover, there is no way a patient will share their deepest fears and darkest secrets with you if you haven't established a trusting therapeutic relationship with them, and they certainly won't be willing to take risks in therapy (like exposure therapy) if they don't trust the therapist's expertise, compassion, and care. My hope is that these case examples will both inform and inspire your care for these patients.

Please note that some of the patient dialog contains profanity. This is intentional. Patients often want to use profanity in session, and are often

DOI: 10.4324/9781003454380-10

relieved when I express comfort with that and "give them permission." Sometimes I use profanity myself, if I know the patient is comfortable with it. I point out that profanity is sometimes the only way to communicate the intensity or depth of feeling a person is experiencing. If you find it offensive, then by all means, set different norms and standards in your own work with patients. I have tried to capture what feels like authentic dialog with patients, and these protocols are pretty good examples of the kinds of things that actually get said in therapy.

Positionality Statement

I want to begin this section by acknowledging that I am a white, straight, married, cis-gendered woman. I am ethnically Jewish on my mother's side, but I consider myself a humanist atheist. I am hearing impaired, but not deaf. I am disfigured by burn and skin graft scars, but I can mostly hide them strategically under clothes. I grew up with a *lot* of white, thin, wealthy, educated privilege as the only child of upper middle class parents who worked as university professors. But I also have some intersectional components to my identity, including being a woman, being hearing impaired, and being disfigured. These cases are of necessity written through the lens of these various aspects of my identity, since that is my lived experience of moving through the world and doing this work. I have done my best to include examples of working with patients from a number of backgrounds, including some with minoritized or racialized identities or low socioeconomic status. The therapist in each case does their best to be aware, self-reflective, and culturally responsive, but inevitably gets things wrong from time to time. I hope that my portrayal of these issues is thought provoking, and provides a useful model for how to think about intersectionality in the context of therapy, especially for therapists who hold white privilege. I do not, however, claim to get things "right." If you are a therapist who holds a minoritized or racialized identity, I ask you to forgive me for not including the experiences of therapists who share your identity. There are, of course, both unique advantages and challenges to doing this work for people from all backgrounds. I can only capture the truth of what I have experienced.

Case 1–Chris

Chris is a 23 year old, white, single, straight cis-man who is a recent college graduate. He has been living at home and working at his father's business to save money while he looks for a job in his chosen field of non-profit environmental work. Chris grew up in a fairly rural small town and has deep ties to his extended family, his church and the broader community. His Crohn's disease was diagnosed relatively early (in late middle school) by the family's gastroenterologist (the only GI doc in their area) because Chris's father also suffers from Crohn's, so he knew to be on the lookout for it. Chris's mom experimented with a number of different dietary approaches to help her husband and son, and the family finally settled on a strict Specific Carbohydrate Diet, which they all believe has been extremely helpful. Chris's mom is a good cook and enjoyed inventing numerous recipes consistent with the diet's guidelines. She appreciates that the overall low carbohydrate diet helps keep her slender. Chris had several years in college of good health living in an apartment and cooking for himself. But the summer after graduation he went on a church mission trip for several months to a South American country. While there, he had much less control over his diet, and also wanted to eat the local cuisine and not think about Crohn's "for once in my life." He started to feel ill during the second month, and by the time he returned home was having frequent abdominal pain and some urgent diarrhea. Now he is back on steroids and is feeling frustrated and very sad about his health. Chris's mom found the therapist online and set up the appointment for him, but he attends by himself via telehealth.

Session 1

Session 1 focuses on taking his history and establishing goals for treatment. The therapist sets the agenda and tells Chris that this is basically an opportunity for them to get to know him, and that they want to save ten minutes at the end to teach him deep diaphragmatic breathing. Initially unsure what help talk therapy can be, he ends up filling almost the entire hour with recounting his history. One thing it turns out he is frustrated about is that the family GI doctor doesn't actually have all that much expertise in IBD. He wonders if his care has really been all that well managed. He's been on steroids on and off for many years, and was on Humira for a short time in high school. The GI doc was a bit dismissive of the dietary restrictions that the family followed, which frustrated Chris and his mom, but they understood that there wasn't a lot of scientific "evidence" to support the diet. The GI doc also ordered bi-monthly iron infusions for him for years to address what appeared to be chronic iron deficiency anemia. Chris is starting to wonder whether he should consult with a new doctor, but feels very ambivalent about "betraying" the doctor who has taken care of their family for so many years, and who continues to care for Chris's dad. He also doesn't want to "make waves" in the family (or their tight knit community) and is unsure how to go about finding a new doctor. He has always relied on his mom to manage his health care decisions, and doesn't want to appear to be second guessing her or questioning her judgment. He would like to get off the steroids and expresses his commitment to returning to a strict Specific Carbohydrate Diet. Approaching the end of the hour he is still telling the story of his time on the mission trip, his host family, the wonderful food they ate, how much he enjoyed the trip and felt inspired by it to include a focus on environmental justice and sustainability in his career. The therapist gently interrupts and tells Chris they need to save a few minutes to learn DDB. Chris looks startled and says "Wait, the whole hour is almost up? Wow, I didn't realize how much I had to talk about! Sorry for not letting you get a word in edgewise." The therapist assures Chris that this is very common, and that lots of people with IBD need to tell their story. Then they teach Chris DDB. He majored in environmental science in college, and is really interested to learn about respiratory sinus arrhythmia and heart rate variability. He wears a fitness watch, and is amazed at how much the DDB changes his heart rate over the course of just one minute. He agrees to practice DDB during the coming week.

Having heard most of Chris's history, the therapist has started to formulate a case conceptualization, but is still unsure about several things. Chris appears to be generally well adjusted, and does not seem to suffer from any psychiatric comorbidities. They consider whether Chris might meet criteria for ARFID, based on his commitment to a highly restrictive diet, but reject the idea. Following the diet does not seem to cause Chris any distress or disability. He may or may not be chronically iron deficient, but that could easily be the result of Crohn's that hasn't been medically managed aggressively enough. Chris seems to be faced with a fairly common developmental challenge for youth with IBD of entering adulthood and taking over management of his own health care moving forward. There are clearly some family system (and even community system) issues that make him feel ambivalent about this, but he is relatively clear eyed about the need. It seems he mostly needed to tell his story, and may need help thinking through how to transition to adulthood and how much "space" to let Crohn's occupy in his life.

Session 2

Chris reports that he enjoyed the deep breathing a lot and feels like he has gotten really good at it. He had a job interview with a non-profit environmental consulting firm that he was nervous about, and he reports that doing five minutes of DDB before the interview started was "amazing" and really left him feeling calm and centered. He's pretty sure he aced the interview, because they have already invited him back for a second round. He is planning to travel out of state for the second interview to the major metropolitan area where the job would be located, and is considering trying to get a consultation with a new GI doc at a large academic medical center that is located there. The therapist praises Chris warmly for doing the homework, and validates his enthusiasm for the potential job, *and* for the idea of securing a consultation with an IBD expert.

Most of the second session is taken up with filling out the rest of his history and discussing how to talk to his mom about switching his care to a new doctor. Chris dated casually in college, and never had trouble explaining his "weird" diet to potential girlfriends. He didn't much like it when a girl tried to express too much concern about his health—"I have my mom for that" he noted. But he acknowledges that eventually he will want a partner who is supportive, without feeling sorry for him. He doesn't want the Crohn's to be "that big a deal" in his life and other than diet, would prefer not to think about it too much. The therapist articulates the basic dilemma here—Crohn's is indeed a chronic disease that will probably need proactive management for the rest of his life. He can't ignore it. He needs to be smart and responsible about his care, getting the periodic diagnostic tests he will need and assembling a medical team he trusts and feels comfortable with. On the other hand, he doesn't want the Crohn's to be center stage in his life, or to define his identity. Chris immediately agrees that that encapsulates the dilemma pretty well. They agree that trying to set up the consultation with a new doctor makes a good deal of sense. Chris's homework is to call the center and secure the appointment.

Session 3

Session 3 takes place three weeks later. Chris reports that he did indeed travel to the other city and that he was offered the job on the spot at the end of the interview. He is thrilled, although he hasn't actually gotten all the information yet about salary and, importantly, health care benefits. He is starting to think through the complexities of managing his disease on his own, and realizes that really good health insurance is going to be crucial for him moving forward. He is considering staying on his family's plan until he is 26, but realizes that may not work well if he is in a different state with different medical networks. The therapist celebrates the job offer, and praises him for considering the importance of health insurance. They agree that it is no fun for a 23 year old to have to think about stuff like that, but that it is a good sign about his transition to adulthood.

More distressingly, Chris shares that he was indeed able to secure a consultation with a true IBD expert at the major medical center. (This was something of a miracle, actually, since the expert is usually booked out many months in advance. But they had a cancelation and they were able to squeeze him in.) The new doctor was a bit horrified by how his care had been managed, especially the reliance on steroids and frequent iron infusions. She sent him for further testing right there and then. This center had access to advanced ultrasonography machines, which allowed her to establish fairly quickly that he was experiencing moderate inflammation and had a few strictures that might or might not resolve with better medication management. She wants to start him on a trial of Stelara as soon as possible. She was actually more concerned about his liver than anything else, and sent him for an MRI that same day. It turns out that years of (unnecessary) chronic, indiscriminate use of iron infusions left him with iron overload. Unchecked, this can lead to fibrosis of the liver or even cirrhosis. Chris is feeling both angry and resigned. He understands that his family GI doctor did the best he could to keep him healthy, but he is also realizing how poorly managed his care has actually been. He is concerned about whether his dad's care is being well enough managed, but he also doesn't want to second guess his parents or cause a rift in their relationship with the doctor "who saved both of our lives" by getting the diagnosis right early on. He also worries about the impact in their tight knit community. Both his dad and the GI doctor serve as deacons in their church. He worries about causing tension, or worse, spreading dissension. He doesn't want to "throw my doctor under the bus" but he also doesn't know what to do with his frustration and anger about the possibility of liver damage. "Like having Crohn's wasn't bad enough!" he says.

The therapist listens and validates both his anger and his ambivalence about calling the doctor out. They suggest that Chris consider writing a letter to the doctor—actually two versions of the letter—neither of which he will actually send. The first letter should focus on his anger—just let it all out on the page. Use strong language or even profanity if it feels like the only way to convey the strong feelings. The second letter should focus on his gratitude for all the years of care he received, and the doctor's important place in his life, in their family and in their community. Once all of that is down on paper, they tell Chris that he may be in a better position to process the complexity of the two narratives, and may see his way to letting the doctor know about the recent findings. After all, it may be that the doctor will feel badly about his mistakes and will be quite open to learning and expanding his expertise on IBD management.

Session 4

Chris reports that he wrote both letters and felt much better afterwards. He had a long conversation with his parents about what to do, and they agreed that it made sense to let the family doctor know about the recent test results. They would thank him for his long term support of Chris and let him know that Chris would be moving for his new job. He would need his records transferred to the new GI doctor. Chris feels good about this decision. His mom shares his anger and concern for his dad's care moving forward, but Chris realizes that that is not his problem to manage. He's feeling a bit of trepidation about starting a new medication regimen. He is also a little freaked out about having to learn to give himself shots (his mom gave him the Humira back in high school), but he is hopeful that a more aggressive medication approach will quickly bring his Crohn's back under control, and that he will figure it out and take it in stride. The therapist recommends that he connect with a Crohn's and Colitis Foundation support group in his area, or use their peer to peer support line to learn tips and tricks for doing the injections. He doesn't much like the idea of a support group—"I don't want to sit around in some random church basement for an hour every month complaining about Crohn's," but he thinks a few chats with an experienced peer via video or phone might indeed be helpful. He is looking forward to moving and starting his new job, and he is generally optimistic about his prospects in life. He and the therapist agree that he has done good work in therapy, and that he doesn't really need any further sessions. He is grateful, and says "I guess I really did need to talk this all through, huh? Thanks for your help. It was nice I didn't have to explain it all to you." The therapist praises him for his thoughtful approach and encourages him to reach out in the future if it ever feels like further support would be useful.

Case 2–Chantal

Chantal is a 24 year old, engaged, African American, straight cis-woman who is working toward her master's degree in elementary education and student teaching in a local school system. She loves working with the kids and she has gotten great feedback from her mentor teacher and the school principal. But Chantal has been struggling with what will ultimately be diagnosed as ulcerative colitis for some months. She has been suffering from frequent bouts of burning abdominal pain and diarrhea when the urge to defecate comes on her so suddenly and powerfully, she is never sure she'll make it to the bathroom on time. It's manageable when it happens at home and she can simply run to the bathroom. But she fears having an attack when she is working with the kids at school or when she is trapped in a class in her master's program. She went to her primary care doctor numerous times. First, he recommended that she eat more fiber. That made her symptoms worse. Then he recommended using anti-diarrheal medications like Imodium. That helped a little, but eventually the pain and diarrhea came back, accompanied by occasional mucus and blood in her stools. She started to feel fatigued, her joints started to hurt, and she stopped running—an activity she used to love. Despite not exercising as much, she lost some weight. It was hard to put back on since she wasn't very hungry and had started to be afraid of the pain that might follow eating. Her doctor shrugged his shoulders and told her she probably had irritable bowel syndrome and that there wasn't much that could be done except avoiding stress or trying various elimination diets, like limiting gluten or dairy. She felt dismissed and strongly suspected that there was racial bias at play, because it felt like the doctor just wasn't taking her seriously.

One night, she woke up in so much pain her fiancé insisted on taking her to the ER. They couldn't find anything wrong, other than a very low grade fever, low iron levels, and an elevated white count in her blood work. They prescribed an antibiotic and sent her home, but they did also strongly suggest a consultation with a gastroenterologist. The new doctor ran a number of tests and discovered that Chantal was not only anemic, she was also deficient in several important vitamins, including B12. He also found blood in her stool, and inflammatory markers in her stool and blood. The gastroenterologist had her schedule an MRE (magnetic resonance enterography) and a colonoscopy. Two weeks later, after all that testing, she finally had a diagnosis: ulcerative colitis. It was nice to know what was actually wrong, but now she wonders if she will ever be able to finish her program, much less work full time as a teacher. She is devastated by the diagnosis, fearful of the long term implications, and is thinking about breaking things off with her fiancé. She is also furious at her primary care doctor for dismissing her symptoms. Suddenly the happy, fulfilling, productive life she envisioned for herself just doesn't seem possible anymore.

Session 1

Chantal has just recently been diagnosed with ulcerative colitis. She is feeling overwhelmed and hopeless, and really wonders if she will be able to continue in her career (which she loves) or to make a life with her fiancé (whom she adores). She has lost weight and has been feeling so fatigued, sore, and ill that she has stopped exercising. It is all she can do to show up for her classes and her student teaching. In the first session, a CBT therapist takes a thorough history, including eliciting information about family of origin, social and academic development, and history of psychiatric symptoms and diagnoses in her family and in Chantal herself. She has always been a happy, healthy, well-adjusted individual, but she is currently experiencing a number of symptoms of depression that don't quite meet criteria for a major depressive disorder. She is also anxious and overwhelmed about all the decisions she feels she has to make. She's having difficulty getting to sleep at night because she lies in bed with her thoughts racing. In light of all this, the best diagnosis appears to be an adjustment disorder with mixed anxious and depressed mood. Indeed, the very fact that she has always been so healthy seems to be a risk factor for adjustment at the moment. Apart from the normal coughs, colds, and occasional stomach bugs of childhood and adolescence, and a serious sprained ankle when she was running track competitively in high school, Chantal has never really had to deal with serious medical issues before. She is convinced that this diagnosis spells the end of all her hopes and plans for a fulfilling life, and it makes her feel quite panicky when she thinks about it.

The therapist secures Chantal's consent to consult with the gastroenterologist to ensure that the therapist is fully informed about the extent of Chantal's illness and the steps the gastroenterologist plans to take to manage it. Chantal is actually quite grateful that the therapist is willing to do this. She wants someone else to help her navigate the complexities of this, and she admits that she tends to feel anxious when talking to doctors and sometimes can't even think of what questions to ask as she tries to absorb what the doctor is saying. She also worries about experiencing further racial bias and feels enormous pressure to be as calm as possible while also ensuring that her concerns are taken seriously. "I don't want him to see me as an 'angry black woman,' even though I *am* angry that my regular doctor wrote me off."

First, the therapist validates Chantal's anger and frustration over her experiences of racial bias from medical professionals, and agrees that the weight of systemic racism in medicine is a lot to navigate. "I'm so sorry that you have to deal with this in addition to everything else you're trying to manage. I will do my best to be an effective ally for you. And even though I will do my best, I may well do or say something at some point that feels clueless or even hurtful. Please know that if you choose to tell me when that happens, I will do my utmost to own it, to apologize and to learn from it." Note that the therapist does *not* question Chantal's perception of her prior doctor's racial bias. Whether or not that individual doctor would have said the exact same thing to a white patient, while certainly possible, is irrelevant. Chantal brought a lifetime of lived experience with systemic racism and microaggressions to that encounter, and the therapist is well aware of the empirical literature documenting racial disparities in health outcomes and especially pain management for African American women. The only appropriate response is validation. As Ijeoma Oluo writes in her excellent book *So You Want to Talk About Race*, something is about race "if a person of color thinks it's about race."[1] It is not that people of color always interpret things correctly and never make assumptions that might be faulty. But it is the case that people of color bring their lived experience and their racial (and cultural) identity to every single interaction they have in the world, and will necessarily experience the world through that lens.

With Chantal's consent, the therapist next moves on to do some basic psychoeducation, and assures Chantal that the vast majority of UC patients live full, rich lives, and that there is no need to give up on her hopes and dreams. Chantal expresses relief at this, although she is still uncertain how she's going to cope with the physical challenges and the treatment protocols. She has never liked taking medication—not even Tylenol, and is very reluctant to fill the prescription for mesalamine that the gastroenterologist gave her. The therapist talks through some of her concerns, and points out that the medication acts primarily in the colon to reduce inflammation, and that it should begin to provide her some symptomatic relief relatively quickly, and

[1] Oluo, I. (2019). *So You Want to Talk About Race,* page 25. Seal Press; New York, NY.

will allow the tissues in her gut to start healing. In fact, it has a good chance of inducing remission. Chantal raises concerns about the possibility of having to stay on the drug if she ever wanted to get pregnant. The therapist smiles and points out how quickly her perspective has shifted. When she started the session, she seemed convinced that she would never be able to marry, and now she's worrying about getting pregnant! Chantal also smiles, and admits that she is already feeling less anxious knowing that someone will be with her to walk her through this journey.

The therapist then explains how anxiety exacerbates some of the physical symptoms Chantal experiences through sympathetic nervous system arousal and assures Chantal that although these sensations are extremely uncomfortable, they are not dangerous. In fact, it is the body reacting normatively to a perceived threat. If the threat were a saber-toothed tiger, the body's "panicky" reaction (increasing respiration and heart rate, secreting adrenaline and cortisol, converting glycogen to glucose, and shutting down digestion) would be quite adaptive! The therapist then teaches Chantal deep diaphragmatic breathing to show her that she has some control over sympathetic versus parasympathetic arousal. Chantal likes this exercise. Although she has recently felt like her body was betraying her, as a former competitive athlete she has always enjoyed practicing physical skills, and she gets the hang of it pretty quickly.

The therapist also reviews some basic insomnia management (cognitive behavioral therapy for insomnia or CBTi) strategies. Like most people, when she can't sleep, Chantal stays in bed thinking it is better to at least "rest" even if she can't sleep. She is surprised when the therapist tells her this is a terrible idea! The therapist explains that staying in bed when you're anxious and frustrated about not being able to sleep just ends up creating an association between bed and anxious arousal—the opposite of what you need to fall asleep. Instead, if she's having trouble sleeping, she should get up, go to a different room, and do something quiet and boring (NOT watching an electronic screen like the TV, phone, or iPad) until she feels sleepy. Then get back into bed and see if sleep overtakes her. Chantal's homework is to practice deep breathing three to four times a day for one minute at a time, at a rate of four breaths per minute, and to get out of bed if she is having trouble falling asleep.

Between Sessions 1 and 2 the therapist calls the gastroenterologist to consult about the case. The doctor informs the therapist that Chantal has what appears to be a fairly mild case of UC that has been caught relatively early. Although it is impossible to know for certain, the doctor is fairly sure that she will respond to first-line treatment with mesalamine. He also offered her a course of budesonide to help her feel better fairly quickly, but Chantal had declined. The doctor notes that he is surprised to hear that Chantal is so anxious and distressed about the diagnosis. He thought she seemed quite calm, took it all in stride and that he had been quite reassuring and encouraging about her prognosis. He appreciates the heads up from the therapist and says he will reach out to her through the patient portal to encourage her to ask any questions she might have and to assure her that he wants to address any concerns or worries that she has.

Session 2

Session 2 begins with a review of the homework. Chantal reports that she practiced the deep breathing a few times a day. She likes it, and says it feels quite helpful, especially at night in bed when she is trying to relax and get to sleep. She has actually thought about incorporating it into a lesson plan for the kids she is student teaching. "It seems like it might be a great way to help them slow down and relax before tackling a difficult lesson." She only got out of bed one night when she had trouble winding down enough to sleep. She felt a little silly, but admitted that after sitting on the couch reading a magazine for about 20 minutes, she got sleepy, went back to bed, and fell right to sleep. She has been getting slightly better sleep and is feeling less exhausted overall, although she still feels quite fatigued and her joints still hurt. The therapist praises Chantal's use of these new skills, and agrees that teaching her students deep breathing is a great idea.

Chantal then confides that she still hasn't started taking the mesalamine. "I keep thinking I ought to be able to get this under control without needing medication," she says. The therapist strongly encourages Chantal to follow her doctor's advice on this score. She tells Chantal about her communication with the doctor, and that the doctor very much wants to hear from her about any concerns she has. She reminds Chantal that UC is an autoimmune disorder, and unless she can magically control her immune system in a way that other human beings can't, she really should take the medication. The therapist reiterates that mesalamine is considered the first-line treatment for UC, and that for many people it will induce remission, symptomatically, endoscopically, and histologically. The therapist then proceeds to help Chantal identify her main goals of treatment. Chantal makes clear that she wants her life back. She wants to teach and get married and have a family of her own. The thing she fears most is that she won't be able to do these things, or that she will end up being a burden on her fiancé, Darius. Keeping these goals in mind, the therapist encourages Chantal to think through how taking the medication will be an important part of helping her achieve these goals. The healthier she is, the more likely she will be to be a successful teacher and an equal partner and parent. Chantal agrees to start taking the medication as prescribed.

At this point in the session, Chantal became quiet and tearful. The therapist probed gently to ask what she was thinking about. She shared that her relationship with Darius has been quite strained over the last month. She has been doing her best to soldier through and take care of things by herself because she doesn't want to depend on him or make him take care of her. She's also embarrassed about her symptoms and has tried to hide her frequent bathroom visits from him, preferring to cancel their plans if she feels like her gut is acting up. He has been alternately understanding and frustrated, especially when she cancels their plans at the last minute. "He's such a great guy—he deserves to be with someone who won't be sick all the time," she says.

The therapist asks Chantal more about her fiancé and the history of their relationship. It seems clear that Darius is, indeed, a great guy, who is committed to the relationship and very much wants to help her navigate the challenges of her illness. The therapist wonders whether perhaps Darius might actually be hurt that she is shutting him out. She asks Chantal to consider how she would feel if the situation were reversed—if Darius had been diagnosed with UC instead of her. Chantal sees instantly that she would want to know everything and would want to help in any way she could—"That's what a good marriage should be, you know, in sickness and in health. I would want to take care of him." The therapist gently points out that by shutting Darius out she is actually hurting their relationship and moving farther away from the trust and intimacy she wants. She agrees that even though it makes her nervous, she will talk to Darius about everything this weekend, and will be more honest with him moving forward. "I don't have to tell him about my bloody poop, though, do I? That seems like a real mood killer." The therapist laughingly agrees that that level of detail right off the bat might be a bit much, but that eventually in a marriage, even bloody poop is something you can talk about.

Session 3

Chantal is pleased to announce at the beginning of the session that she has started taking the mesalamine as prescribed, and isn't noticing any weird side effects, but isn't feeling any better yet either. The therapist encourages Chantal to stick with it, and reminds her that it can take two to six weeks to start feeling better, so she shouldn't feel discouraged. The therapist also reminds Chantal that she needs to tell her gastroenterologist when she actually started taking it, so that they can accurately track her response to the medication. Chantal admits to some anxiety about doing this. "I'm afraid the doctor will be frustrated with me and think I'm a bad patient. I don't want to give him any reason to write me off." The therapist reiterates how important it is to have open, honest communication with her gastroenterologist, and strongly encourages Chantal to use the online chart system to let her doctor know that she has now started the medication as prescribed.

Chantal also shares that she talked to Darius over the weekend. She was surprised at how hurt he had been by her efforts to "protect" him and not depend on him. "He said he *wants* me to be able to depend on him. Otherwise what's the point!? He pointed out that the whole 'strong black woman' stereotype is just racist bullshit left over from slavery and of *course* he wants to take care of me and have me lean on him. I realized that shutting him out was a mistake. He felt like it meant I didn't trust him. Of course I trust him! I actually feel a lot closer to him now." The therapist praises Chantal warmly for being brave enough to talk to Darius honestly about her fears and her symptoms. She also invites Chantal to talk through how the "strong black woman" stereotype has impacted her in her life. "We're supposed to be able to handle everything, you know? Just absorb the pain and deal with it and be there for everyone else. Kind of self-sacrificing and not having needs or emotions of our own. Darius is right. It's racist bullshit." Chantal pauses for a moment, and then continues "It has its origins in the idea that enslaved black women didn't feel pain and could labor all day like beasts of burden—look it up sometime." The therapist expresses interest and some surprise about this, and admits to Chantal that they always thought of "strong black woman" as a compliment. They thank Chantal for explaining it, and say they can see how harmful the stereotype could be to both the black community and to individual black women. They also promise to do some research on their own and educate themselves further about it.

The therapist then asks if they can address the issue of how shame and secrecy were driving Chantal's decisions about what to tell Darius and explains that shame and secrecy can make the burdens associated with GI disorders a lot worse. To further this point, the therapist asks what, if anything, Chantal has shared with her mentor teacher, the principal at the school, and her preceptor in her master's program. Chantal looks at the therapist like the *therapist* is crazy and says "Nothing! Why would I want to tell them what I'm dealing with? Okay, I get why Darius needed to know, but not my co-workers who are supervising and judging me and my work." "I'm really worried they see me as unreliable or flaky—which is bad enough if you're white—but the last thing I want is to give anyone an excuse to think I'm lazy or irresponsible. I've just needed so many sick days over the last few months." The therapist validates Chantal's concerns about the double standard that many people of color experience – needing to work twice as hard to achieve the same level of recognition, but then guides Chantal to think through how stressful it is at work when she needs to use the bathroom but feels she can't step away from the class. The therapist encourages Chantal to be honest with her co-workers. Chantal looks quite skeptical about this, but agrees to tell just her mentor teacher some of the basic facts of what she's been dealing with.

Session 4

Chantal is pleased to report that she told her mentor teacher about her UC and was pleasantly surprised that the senior teacher was not only sympathetic, she was pleased that Chantal had shared the truth with her. The senior teacher *had* been worried that Chantal wasn't really committed to teaching, despite her excellent work with the students when she was there, and was actually relieved to learn that Chantal had been coping with a specific medical issue and had simply been too embarrassed to tell her the truth. In a twist of fate, it turns out that the senior teacher's niece had been diagnosed with Crohn's disease at age 16, and the teacher was familiar with IBD and everything they entailed. Now that the teacher knows the truth, the two of them have come up with some strategies to manage it if Chantal does need to step out to use the bathroom. As a result, Chantal feels more confident about going in to teach even if her gut is acting up a bit in the morning, and she hasn't missed a day all week. She does admit, however, that she never eats breakfast or lunch on school days, to minimize the chances that she will need to run to the bathroom.

In light of the progress she has made, the therapist encourages Chantal to stop skipping breakfast and lunch. The therapist has Chantal consider the effects of hunger on her mood, concentration, and energy. Indeed, she gets Chantal to acknowledge that when her students are irritable, reactive, distractible, and tired it is often because they are hungry! Chantal agrees to try eating a small "safe" breakfast of soluble fiber rich oatmeal and a few blueberries or half a banana. With the "okay" from the gastroenterologist, Chantal also knows that she can take some anti-diarrheal medication on days when her gut is acting up. Overcoming her resistance to using any medication at all is somewhat challenging. Once again, the therapist reminds Chantal of her central goals and values. If the goal is to be an attentive, patient, effective teacher, then neither being hungry (and impatient and irritable) or needing to run to the restroom frequently are ideal. Using anti-diarrheal medication judiciously and appropriately can be an important part of managing her symptoms and allowing her to achieve her goals. Chantal admits that her doctor told her it was fine to use anti-diarrheal medication if she needed it, and that she will try it this week.

Session 5

Chantal is pleased to report that she ate breakfast every day this week, and did indeed feel more focused, had more energy, and felt quicker on her feet during her lessons. She used an anti-diarrheal medication three of the four days she was in the classroom and it did feel helpful. She actually didn't poop at all on day three, so she stopped taking the medication after that, and then had a normal bowel movement on the fifth day, followed by a return of some diarrhea thereafter. She notes that the burning pain seems to be lessening, and she hasn't noticed any mucus or blood in her stool all week. The therapist points out that this is good news, and that perhaps the mesalamine is starting to take effect. Chantal admits that she is feeling better and that getting through the day is starting to feel a bit more normal. She does admit that she still doesn't eat lunch on school days, partly because she is so busy and partly because she is afraid of bringing on symptoms. The therapist encourages her to try to fit in at least a small snack every day, pointing out that teaching is an intense job, and that all teachers need to learn to protect their own work-life balance and engage in appropriate self-care.

Chantal is still anxious about experiencing pain or feeling an urgent need to move her bowels during a class or during staff meetings, and she is very anxious about the upcoming parent–teacher conferences, which meet back to back for three hours without a break. While the senior teacher is primarily responsible for these, Chantal is expected to take part as well. Chantal is also anxious about an upcoming evaluation, in which her preceptor from her program will be observing her teach for an afternoon. The therapist encourages her to identify her catastrophic thoughts, and then replace them with more realistic, benign beliefs.

Session 6

Chantal reports that she got through the parent–teacher conferences successfully and notes that she was so busy and focused on what she needed to convey about each child, that she actually didn't think about her gut at all. Her live evaluation went well. She felt somewhat crampy and uncomfortable that morning, so she did use some anti-diarrheal medication that day, but the actual teaching went well and she got through it with flying colors.

She also raises the issue that her cousin is getting married the following weekend, and she is supposed to be a bridesmaid. She is nervous about flying out of state and getting through the entire ceremony and reception. She has never been a nervous flier in the past, but now the thought of being trapped in her seat on the airplane and then being around all her extended family (and all the strangers on her cousin's fiancé's side of the family) is making her feel like she should just cancel the whole trip. She is worried about being trapped in her seat on the plane and *needing* to use the toilet. She's also worried about drawing attention to herself if she feels sick during the wedding ceremony or the reception. She loves her aunt, uncle, and cousin, and doesn't want to do anything to detract from their special day. "I don't want to make it about me—what if I get sick and ruin the whole day? I don't want them to hate me!"

The therapist reviews her fears about flying and about her extended family. Together they complete an imaginal exposure exercise in which the therapist walks her through an entire flight in imagination, including using the tiny airplane restroom, some turbulence, the seat belt sign being turned on, and the long wait to deplane at the gate. They also talk through the "worst case scenario" for the wedding and think through how to talk to her cousin in advance. She is able to see that, like shutting Darius out early on, simply canceling the trip and skipping the wedding is not the best option for anyone. She agrees that using anti-diarrheal medication is helpful, and that actually she is starting to feel better and better each week on the mesalamine, so perhaps the wedding trip won't be so difficult after all.

Session 7

Chantal skipped a week of treatment, since she was out of town at her cousin's wedding. She is pleased to report that the whole trip went off without a hitch. She was a little nervous standing in the security line at the airport on the trip out, but once she was on the plane she stayed occupied, reading a magazine, talking to Darius, and even took a short nap. She didn't need to get up even once. The wedding itself was lovely, and she realizes how silly she's been thinking everyone would notice every little thing about her. She did excuse herself from the rehearsal dinner to go to the bathroom, but it was no big deal, and she doesn't think anyone even noticed. She got a little nervous about the drive from the ceremony to the reception. Darius was tasked with driving several elderly relatives and she rode with the other bridesmaid and a groomsman. She felt a few twinges of cramp on the drive, but she was able to breath and tell herself it was no big deal, and the cramps went away. Even if she had had to ask the driver to pull over at a gas station or convenience store so she could go to the bathroom, she realizes it would have been fine. She is thrilled that the flight and the wedding went off so successfully. Her confidence is growing, and she is starting to believe that she can live a normal, full life even with UC. Chantal and the therapist agree that she can wait two weeks for her next session.

Session 8

Chantal reports that, overall, she is pleased with how things are going. She is still anxious about what the future may hold, but she is feeling much more at peace and no longer believes that a teaching career and a life with Darius, including having children, are out of reach.

Chantal shyly confides that now that she is feeling better, she and Darius are making love again. She admits that she had been feeling so ill, so unhappy with her body, and so terrified of experiencing incontinence and soiling the sheets and humiliating herself, that she had stopped having sex with him months ago. She is feeling much more confident about the state of her bowels now. She did have a few concerning thoughts about how her body has changed. She is eating more regularly and has gained back some healthy weight in the time she's been in therapy, but she still feels terribly out of shape and flabby, and was worried that Darius would be totally turned off by her. Not surprisingly, Darius was an enthusiastic participant, and didn't seem the least bit concerned. He just stroked her face and told her how beautiful she was and how much he had missed her. She is thrilled to have that part of her life back.

Darius is now talking about going camping together at a national park, which is making Chantal anxious again. The therapist chimes in assuming that Chantal is simply anxious about bathroom access and makes a somewhat lame joke about pit toilets and outhouses. However, Chantal looks somewhat annoyed and says "That's only a part of it." She goes on to explain that she did not grow up camping at all, and that people of color are dramatically underrepresented at campgrounds and in national parks, and often feel marginalized, unwelcome, or even unsafe in those spaces. The therapist pauses for a moment to reflect, and then apologizes and thanks Chantal for correcting their naive assumption that their camping experiences would be equivalent. It turns out that several years ago Darius discovered the group "Black Folks Camp Too" and has been determined to reclaim the wilderness for himself and for Chantal. They used to hike together regularly, and had some wonderful experiences, but since the onset of her UC she has indeed been too worried about the proximity of bathrooms to risk being out in the woods. The additional pressures of feeling singled out and possibly targeted by hostile white hikers or campground managers makes the whole exercise feel overwhelming. The therapist acknowledges that it never occurred to them that there would be complexities there that they themselves have never experienced, but asks Chantal to reflect on the positive experiences she and Darius had previously. It would be a shame to let her worries about bathroom access get in the way of their enjoyment of this activity. "I do really love being out in nature," Chantal says. "I love the idea of snuggling together by a campfire, looking at the stars—it seems magical. And I know he wants to share that with me." She is feeling much better now physically, and is less anxious overall about her GI symptoms. She decides that she will tell Darius to go ahead and book the campsite. She reflects that two months ago, it would have seemed impossible to even contemplate.

Toward the end of the session, the therapist reviews with Chantal everything she has learned, and confirms that her UC is now under far better control. She still has up to three loose bowel movements a day, but the burning pain and urgency have stopped, and she no longer sees any blood or mucus in her stool. Importantly, she is no longer afraid of experiencing incontinence. Moreover, she now understands that her catastrophic thoughts about what other people would think were distorted and unnecessarily negative. While she doesn't plan on telling everyone she meets that she has a "bloody poop" problem, she is much more comfortable sharing the basic outlines of UC with friends, extended family and co-workers. She is socializing again and has even started eating out—something she hadn't done in months. She is eating more regularly in general and has gained back some of the weight she had lost. She is still a little nervous about expanding her diet, but she is willing to give it a try. Most importantly, she no longer feels overwhelmed by the diagnosis or despairing about her future. She has a good working relationship with her gastroenterologist, and tentatively trusts her doctor to take her seriously and work with her collaboratively. She also understands the importance of being honest with her doctor and managing her care proactively to maximize her quality of life. With the therapist's reassurance that if she feels she needs more support in the future, she can always come back, Chantal decides to terminate therapy and tackle the rest of her issues on her own. She asks the therapist if she can have a hug, and thanks them fervently for "giving me hope for my life back."

Case 3–Julie

Julie is a 27 year old, white, single, straight cis-woman who is currently unemployed and living with her mother, despite being trained and licensed as a dental hygienist. She was diagnosed with Crohn's at the age of 15. Her older brother, who is in his early 30s, also has Crohn's and has at times been extremely ill. He had a resection surgery in his early 20s and ended up with an ostomy for almost a year. Julie is terrified of this happening to her. She started college at age 18, but had a rough go of it and ended up dropping out after her freshman year. She had disability accommodations at school allowing her extended deadlines (in case of illness) and special housing with an en suite bathroom. Unfortunately, she was struggling with so much inflammation, pain, and urgency that her physician insisted on enteral feeding with an NG tube. The tube was placed by a nurse, and Julie hooked herself up to liquid nutrition through the tube at night. Unfortunately, she was not given the option of removing and replacing the tube herself, so she had to leave it in, taped to her cheek where it was highly visible, throughout the day. She made it through her first year this way, but developed such severe depression and social anxiety that she couldn't face returning to school, despite not needing the feeding tube anymore. She still feels "marked" by the stigma of having worn the tube as a freshman. Eventually she was able to attend a local community college that offered an associate's degree in dental hygiene. She graduated from the program, and passed the licensing exam, but has yet to seek employment in her field. She is struggling with significant social anxiety, depression, ongoing fatigue and anemia, and moderate abdominal pain and constipation.

Session 1

As usual, Session 1 involves establishing a relationship, taking a history, and teaching DDB. Julie's narrative focuses alternately on the challenges of her Crohn's and her low self-esteem. Lovely, sweet, and waifish, she is currently significantly underweight, pale, fatigued, and chronically constipated. She is also depressed, socially anxious, and struggling with self-confidence. She feels overwhelmed by the thought of looking for a job, but also feels developmentally paralyzed. "All my high school friends graduated college and have great jobs. Some of them are married and starting to have kids. I'm so stuck. But I feel so awful all the time. I'm exhausted and weak and I feel sick. I can't concentrate on anything for very long. I can't imagine applying for jobs or trying to work. And I've probably already forgotten everything I need to know."

Presented with a range of severe problems, the therapist has to decide where to focus this first session. Because it may be difficult to disentangle the source of Julie's exhaustion and demoralization, the therapist decides to focus on Crohn's management and diet first. Fatigue, concentration difficulties, and lack of motivation could be due to depression, but they could also be due to underlying disease and malnutrition. The therapist asks Julie to allow them to consult with Julie's GI doctor, to which she readily agrees. The therapist also inquires about Julie's day to day schedule and diet. Julie is doing very little—mostly just lying on the couch. She tries to get up a few times a day to play with her dog, but doesn't have the energy to walk the dog outside the house. It turns out she is living almost entirely on peanut butter and jelly sandwiches on white bread. The therapist notes that this is not a complete diet, and that it is no wonder Julie is severely constipated and tired all the time. They strongly suggest that Julie ask for bloodwork to check on iron and B12 levels.

The therapist then turns to getting a more complete psychosocial history. Julie's freshman year of college was fairly traumatizing, and did nothing to help her overcome her social anxiety. "Lots of people just assumed I had an eating disorder—like anorexia. I wore the feeding tube, and I was really thin. I think a lot of people just shied away from me. I was kind of marked as 'that crazy anorexic girl.' The only people who were willing to take the trouble to get to know me were other girls with issues. It was cool that I had people to hang out with, but I'm not friends with any of them anymore. They were a pretty high drama crowd." The therapist empathizes with Julie's situation and remarks on how surprised they are that she wore a 24/7 feeding tube for enteral feeding at the age of 18–19. Her Crohn's is more stable now, and she is maintained on Remicade infusions every six weeks. But her highly restricted diet is still obviously problematic.

Julie recounts having a better time at her dental hygiene program than she did her freshman year, but notes that many of the girls were younger than she was and she didn't really feel like she had much in common with any of them. It was also a commuter school, so there were few opportunities to cultivate close friendships. Julie acknowledges that she did well academically in her program and on her clinical rotations, and passed the licensing exam on the first try. But she hasn't touched any of her notes or study guides since, and is worried that she is no longer up to speed on the technical aspects of her field. "My mom and grandparents helped me pay for the program, and I feel so guilty that I'm not using my degree."

The therapist spends some time talking to Julie about what her goals are for treatment. Julie says that of course she would love to be healthy and working full time and living in her own apartment and making friends and even dating eventually, but then she tears up and says quietly "but none of that seems possible to me. I have no idea how to even get started."

The therapist agrees that it might seem daunting, but that they are confident they can help Julie accomplish all of these things. The first steps will be to learn to manage acute anxiety a bit better with DDB, to check on her nutritional status, and to start improving her diet. If she starts to feel better, she might find that she could start reintroducing physical activity and exercise, which will be important since dental hygiene work requires physical stamina. Julie's homework is to practice DDB during the week, to which she readily agrees.

Session 2

Between sessions the therapist called the GI doc to confer. The doctor readily agreed to order labs and said they would be happy to see if Julie's insurance company would approve an iron infusion if necessary. The doctor was horrified to learn that she has been subsisting on PBJ sandwiches, and assures the therapist that there is no medically warranted reason for such a restricted diet.

When Julie attends the second session, she tells the therapist that she already got the lab work done and that she is in fact both anemic and B12 deficient. She has started taking a sublingual B12 supplement, and is hoping to get an iron infusion the following week. The therapist praises Julie for getting this done and points out that much of her exhaustion and cognitive fatigue might actually be the result of these deficiencies. Once they are addressed, she might start to feel significantly better. The therapist then raises the question of Julie's diet. Julie has always preferred a vegetarian diet for ethical and moral reasons, but she is also lactose intolerant and doesn't drink cow's milk. She does like eggs, in theory. The therapist agrees that eggs are a wonderful source of complete protein, but also encourages her to start adding some fiber back into her diet. Since she has been struggling with constipation, the therapist recommends switching to whole wheat bread, and adding soluble fiber from fruits and a few vegetables, like zucchini, sweet potatoes, and squash. Julie is anxious about expanding her diet but agrees that she needs to try. "PBJ is just the only thing that I like and feels safe," she says. But she is willing to have a scrambled egg and to try a smoothie blend with soy milk, banana, and blueberries, since she generally finds sweet things more appealing and soothing. The therapist also encourages her to add Benefiber to her diet to increase the soluble fiber quickly.

The therapist then turns their attention to the need to begin some behavioral activation. It has been very difficult for Julie to do much of anything, given her fatigue, and how demoralized she has been feeling. They agree that it is premature to start exercising, but the therapist suggests spending a little time on job search websites "just to see what's out there." Julie reacts very negatively to this, wailing "What's the point!? I can't possibly interview for a job right now. I have no stamina or strength and I can't remember anything!" The therapist apologizes for jumping ahead, and agrees that looking at job postings might be premature. Instead, they ask Julie what she *does* think she could manage. "I don't know, maybe I could pull out my class notes from anatomy and see if I can start reviewing things. Honestly I don't think I even remember how to label individual teeth right now." The therapist agrees that this would be a good place to start. They remind Julie that this is a process. Eventually achieving her goals will require gradual progress on a number of fronts. Julie's homework is to pull her notebook out and at least look at it.

Session 3

Julie reports that they got the approval for her iron infusion in record time and she had it done earlier that week. "I'm already feeling better," she admits. "I don't get winded going up the stairs and I'm not napping as much in the afternoon. My doctor also gave me a B12 injection. Maybe some of this was just nutritional deficiencies." The therapist is delighted that she has made progress on addressing this with medical management. Julie also reports that she asked her mom to buy some whole wheat bread and has eaten it for the last few days. She also ate a scrambled egg with some toast, and that seemed to sit well. The smoothie was unappealing and she ended up throwing most of it away, but she says she will keep trying. "I might try strawberries instead of banana next time. It was honestly too sweet even for me." She took some Benefiber mixed in with coconut water, and she had a somewhat more normal poop the very next morning. "I guess it worked. It made me really gassy though, which was super uncomfortable." The therapist suggests that she try Citrucel instead, and praises her for being willing to try any of these interventions.

Unfortunately, Julie was unable to get herself to pull out her old school notebook. The therapist problem solves this with her and has her complete a thought record. Julie is able to identify her fear that she will pull out the notes and it will all "look like a foreign language." "What am I going to do if I can't remember anything? It'll be like starting from scratch. I feel so stupid." Together they consider the alternative, which is that she will remember far more than she thinks. "Maybe …" she says tentatively. The therapist then has Julie do a decisional balancing exercise. This helps Julie realize that the reason she's avoiding looking at her notes is that she is terrified she will have forgotten everything and will never be able to get a job. But she sees that *avoiding* looking at her notes (and applying for jobs) *guarantees* that she will never get a job. Given that one of her major goals is to get a full time job so she can afford to get an apartment and move out of her mother's house, it is clear that avoiding reviewing the material moves her farther away from that goal. The therapist encourages her to problem solve what she will do if, indeed, she has forgotten a lot. "Well, I guess I'll just review it. I did pass my licensing exam on the first try. I can't be a total idiot. If I knew it all once, I can learn it again." Julie's homework is, once again, to review her notes and to continue expanding her diet.

Session 4

Julie reports that she did finally get herself to pull her notes out the night before the session. "I didn't want to show up yet again not having done it," she says somewhat chagrined. The therapist assures her that many people do their therapy homework the night before. It just shows that accountability is useful. Julie then explains that although she has certainly forgotten some details, she remembers more than she thought she would. It started to come back to her fairly quickly. She still thinks she is nowhere close to being able to actually interview for a job, but she isn't terrified of studying anymore. The therapist praises her warmly for mustering the courage to confront her fear, and tells her with a smile that they had been quite sure that that would be the outcome.

Julie also shares that she has been walking her dog around the neighborhood at least once a day. Her mom suggested a work out app they could do together that's designed for people who are very out of shape. They tried it together once and had a good laugh about the whole thing. She was a bit appalled by how weak she was. "I can't even hold a plank for 15 seconds—my arms just started to shake." But she is committed to trying to get stronger. "I'll never be able to work even part time if I don't get my strength back." Again the therapist praises Julie for increasing her physical activity.

Julie admits that her mood is improving a *little* with all of this work, but when she actually thinks about working or moving into her own place it still feels completely overwhelming. They continue to work on cognitive reappraisal. Julie becomes tearful quite easily when she thinks about how lonely, isolated, and developmentally "behind" she is. The therapist takes a bit more social and developmental history. It turns out that Julie's dad was quite difficult—arrogant, narcissistic, and often judgmental or even hostile. He frequently criticized both her and her brother for being "difficult" and seemed to scorn them for having medical difficulties. He was often sarcastic, belittling, and even cruel about everything from their looks to their grades in school. "I guess he wanted perfect children that he could be proud of, and we just didn't cut it. I tried so hard to please him, but it never worked. My brother just got mad and cut off contact with him as soon as he left for college, but I kept trying for years." Her parents ultimately divorced and despite her father's wealth (he was a busy real estate lawyer much sought after in the city, with some political aspirations within city government) he was often late with child support and refused to help with college tuition for either of them. "He remarried about eight years ago—some blond socialite. They have two young kids together. I guess he got the family he actually wanted with them. We really don't talk to him at all anymore." The therapist begins to help Julie understand that her father's harsh criticism and lack of loving empathy set the stage for her core schema about being stupid and inept and never good enough. The therapist expresses some anger on Julie's behalf and asks her "Can *you* imagine doing that to a child? A child who is doing their very best despite a serious physical illness? What kind of person does that?"

Julie agrees that her father was pretty horrible, but says it is hard to disentangle what she learned from him versus what her own experiences have taught her. "I *did* basically fail out of college. I managed to get an associate's degree, but I can't work. I can't even remember half of what I learned. I can't support myself. I have no friends. I've never dated seriously. I hate my body.

I'm ugly …" The therapist gently but firmly interrupts this self-loathing litany. "Wow, that is some seriously mean stuff you're telling yourself. Would you ever say any of those things to a friend who was in your position?" "Of course not!" Julie replies. "That would be horrible." "Then why are you saying those things to yourself?" the therapist asks. "It's not helpful to beat yourself up. In fact, how does it make you feel when you say those things?" "Terrible," Julie admits. "And what happens to your self-confidence and your energy and motivation to study your notes and get back in shape and start applying for jobs?" the therapist asks. "Well it all goes in the toilet, so to speak," Julie says. "Right," the therapist replies. "So let's try a new strategy. Let's be realistic about what the challenges are, but let's not allow your father's voice into the room." Julie agrees that this would be a good strategy to try, but she's not sure she knows how to do it. "Well, every time you start having thoughts like that, imagine your father as a tiny little devil on your shoulder whispering those mean hurtful things into your ear. Imagine picking him up by the back of shirt and holding him in front of you and telling him to shut up, and then fling him across the room or out the window. This will help you remember not to internalize that horrible view of yourself." Julie smiles at this idea and says she will give it a shot. Her homework this week is to continue trying to study and exercise and expand her diet bit by bit.

Session 5

Julie reports that she continues to make incremental progress on a number of fronts. She is trying to walk her dog every day and do at least a few strength training sessions every week. She has added a few more fruits and vegetables back into her diet, as well as eggs. She even managed to get to the grocery store herself, rather than relying on her mother to do all the shopping, so that she could see what appealed to her and buy things to make a few dishes she thought she would like. She is still only pooping a few days a week, but is feeling a bit less bloated and uncomfortable and a bit more energetic overall.

She has been reviewing her notes and is trying to build up the courage to call her program director at the community college to ask her for a recommendation and some advice about where to apply. She is still deeply anxious about trying to get a job, and is very worried that her Crohn's will make it very difficult for her to work full time. "What if I have to call in sick? What if I'm so exhausted halfway through the day that my hands start to shake?" She wonders if she should look for a half time position to start with to test the waters. "But I don't know if anyone would hire me for a part time position." The therapist mentions that their own dentist's office has been having trouble scheduling cleanings frequently enough due to turnover and is looking for new staff all the time. Especially post-COVID, many employers are more willing to be flexible. "You can always ask," the therapist encourages her.

This week, Julie mentions that one of her high school friends is having a baby shower and has invited Julie to attend. Julie is deeply ambivalent about this. "I don't know if I can face it. I'm happy for her, but it just feels awful to be around other people who are progressing in their lives when I'm so stuck. It's just embarrassing. Plus I don't have anything to wear. Nothing fits me. I don't know what to say to people if they ask me what I'm up to. 'Nothing!' I guess. How can I face any of those people? I'm so awkward and unsure of myself in the best of circumstances and now I really have nothing to talk about."

The therapist takes this opportunity to educate Julie about social anxiety, shame, the spotlight effect, and cognitive distortions that underlie so much of how she views herself. Julie is objectively a very pretty, sweet young woman. She does come across as a little anxious and fragile at times, and she isn't in a great place in her life, but she is probably dramatically overestimating the degree to which people will be judgmental. The therapist models for Julie how she might talk about her situation at such an event. "I graduated from dental hygiene school at the start of COVID and passed my licensing exam, but it was a terrible time to enter the job market and I was dealing with a Crohn's flare, so I've been working on getting better and I'm planning to start applying for jobs soon." Julie admits that "It doesn't sound so bad when I hear you say it." The therapist points out that it also has the advantage of being true! They practice several iterations of this conversation until Julie feels more comfortable. The therapist points out that loneliness and isolation have been contributing to Julie's depression, and that reaching out to old friends is a good way to try to step back into socializing. She also acknowledges that it's not easy to see people when you're not feeling great about your life. But she encourages Julie to buy one nice outfit for herself and to go to the shower.

Session 6

Julie attended the shower. "I bought a few things and ended up returning them all. Shopping is so demoralizing. I hate it. But then I found an old sundress in my closet that actually looked really cute on me, so I wore that. I felt really awkward at the beginning. Some of those girls were really 'fake' back in high school. But then one girl I really respect got there and we ended up talking for a while. It was really nice. She's really successful but also really down to earth. I forgot how much I like her. She's also still single, which makes it easier. We have plans to get together this weekend to see a movie and get our nails done. I'm actually looking forward to that. It was still really hard though."

The therapist praises Julie for going to the shower and for making plans with a friend, and encourages her to continue reaching out and connecting with people. They then turn their attention to her plans around the job search. She did reach out to her old program director, who was very encouraging and told her there were lots of openings in the region for hygienists. "In a way it's a good time," Julie says. "Being on immunosuppressive medication, I really couldn't have worked in health care at the height of COVID. And lots of other people quit or changed careers, so apparently there are lots of jobs available. She even thinks I could probably find something part time, which would be great. I'm really nervous about whether I have the stamina to work full time yet." The therapist cheers this good news and encourages Julie to start looking at job postings. Julie agrees to try, but then starts worrying about exactly where to look.

"Right now I'm living with my mom, but I don't want to stay there long term. I don't want a long commute either. I don't know whether to look for jobs close to our house, or to look in places where I think I might want to get an apartment." The therapist encourages Julie to look for jobs that are convenient to where she is currently living. "Let's give you time to acclimate to being at work and make sure it's something you can sustain. Then you can save up money over six months and think about the possibility of moving to your own place." Julie agrees that this makes sense. They spend much of the rest of the session de-catastrophizing and problem solving about how Julie will update her resume, how she will talk about the gaps in her schooling and work history during an interview, and so on. Julie's self-esteem remains quite fragile, and the therapist has to say several times "That sounds like your father's voice talking again. Stop being so mean to yourself!"

For the final ten minutes of the session, the therapist has Julie do an imaginal rescripting exercise in which she chooses a specific incident of her father's harsh criticism of her as a child. Together, they imagine Julie's adult self stepping into the memory in order to protect her child self from her father's emotional abuse. The therapist has Julie flip back and forth between seeing the scene from her child perspective and her adult perspective. The therapist helps script what adult Julie would say to her father if she had actually been present to protect her younger self. At the end of the exercise, Julie says "That was weird. I was so scared of him when I was seeing him through my little kid eyes. I'm still kind of scared of him, but I also saw him as just mean and kind of pathetic. Who bullies a little kid? It felt really good to tell him he was an asshole and then tell little Julie that she was strong and brave and resilient and amazing. I hope I can kind of carry that feeling with me."

Session 7

Julie actually had to cancel and reschedule her seventh appointment because she had a job interview. "I couldn't believe it!" she tells the therapist. "I heard back the day after I posted my resume. It's a part time position. They wanted someone to work three ten hour days, but said they might be open to my working five six hour days instead. I think that would be better for me to start with. The hourly pay is pretty good and they said I can shadow someone for the first week to get the hang of their office. They're going to let me know later this week. It happened so fast!" The therapist congratulates Julie on this development, and points out that they have only been working together for two months. "Look how far you've come in such a short time!" Julie acknowledges the therapist's praise, but immediately reverts back to anxious rumination. "Yeah, but I don't actually know if I can do it. They want someone with anesthesia experience—what if I screw up? What if I can't remember the right values or I give the wrong dose? What if I get tired or can't concentrate and I make a mistake and hurt someone?" The therapist points out to Julie how she is anticipating the worst case scenarios, and encourages her to take it one day at a time.

The therapist then suggests that they try some mindfulness meditation exercises. Julie agrees to this, after the therapist explains the rationale. "You get so overwhelmed by anxiety-provoking thoughts and physical sensations, I think this will be a good way to help you distance yourself from your anxiety-provoking thoughts." The therapist leads Julie through a basic series of mindful awareness exercises, gently encouraging her throughout to bring her attention back to the therapist's voice and to the sensations they are choosing to focus on. At the end of the session, Julie opens her eyes and says "Wow. That was really relaxing. My mind started to spin off into anxious thoughts a few times, but I tried to do what you said and just bring it back to the breath, or my heartbeat or the sound of the white noise machine. I can see how that would be useful if I practiced it regularly." Julie's homework is to do just that.

Session 8

Amazingly, Julie got the job. The therapist celebrates with her and congratulates her on this achievement. "It's my first real job," Julie says. "I'm so scared I'm going to screw it up." She is scheduled to start shadowing the following week, and plans to spend the time reviewing her notes and trying to be sure she keeps exercising and stretching. "It's a good thing I can eat a little more normally now," she points out. "There's no way I could do this job if I was barely getting any calories all day long."

The therapist and Julie spend much of this session continuing to do some imaginal rescripting around childhood trauma and focusing on mindfulness skills to help her manage and deflect her anxious, self-defeating thoughts. Julie leaves the session filled with trepidation about starting the position, but determined to try to be professional and capable and make the most of the opportunity.

Sessions 9 and Beyond

Julie is an individual for whom eight sessions was not nearly enough. Although she made substantial progress within this time frame, she still has a long way to go. She still needs to adjust to a new job (which will come with many challenges, tearful sessions, a short time on a performance improvement plan, and lots of coaching by the therapist to be assertive about asking for help and guidance from the senior dentist and other experienced office staff), move to her own apartment, learn to budget, expand her social network and even start tentatively dating. She will deal with Crohn's flares and need to go on and off steroids a few times. At one point she will experience a series of transient bowel obstructions, which the therapist will insist she talk to her doctor about, and her gastroenterologist will recommend surgery. Fearful of taking too much time off of work, she will opt for an endoscopic balloon dilation, which will be helpful, and will buy her time to switch to a new medication. Along the way she will continue to work on her core defectiveness schema and her social anxiety. At the two year mark of therapy, Julie will finally be feeling self-confident enough to "pause" therapy. She will have achieved most of the goals she started therapy with, although she will still be single and only beginning to put a toe in the dating waters. She will also anxiously ask the therapist for reassurance that she can resume treatment if she needs to. The therapist will express confidence in her, but assure her that they will remain available to her "just in case."

Case 4–Arun

Arun is a 28 year old, South Asian Indian, straight, married cis-man. He works as a software developer for a large company. His family is still primarily in India, but he and his sister both attended college in the US. He then stayed on in the US for two years with a STEM OPT visa extension (optional practical training for students in science, technology, engineering, and math). His employer was then able to sponsor him successfully in the lottery for a three year H1B visa (for individuals in specialty or technical occupations) which has already been renewed once and will expire in two years. Arun is married to a white American woman, and they are planning on applying for a green card for him (permanent residence status based on marriage). Unfortunately that process can take several years, and he would be unable to leave the country while waiting for it to be approved. He has aging grandparents in India, and hates the idea of not being able to see them for a long stretch of time, although with his new onset agoraphobia (see below), he wonders if he could even muster the courage to travel to India anyway.

Arun was diagnosed with ulcerative proctitis—a variant of UC that is confined to the anus and rectum—when he was 25. It was well managed for several years with a combination of budesonide and then mesalamine suppositories. Unfortunately, shortly after a routine surveillance colonoscopy when he was 27, he became extremely ill with a hospital acquired *C. diff* (*Clostridioides difficile*) infection. He experienced terrible watery diarrhea, cramping, nausea, vomiting, weakness, and a high fever. His wife drove him to the ER and he was quickly admitted. The hospital gave him supportive treatment (e.g., IVs to minimize dehydration), but it took several rounds of aggressive antibiotic treatment to bring the infection under control, and he felt quite sick for weeks. Ever since that experience, he has developed significant health anxiety and agoraphobia around driving or being too far away from home. Ironically, the thing he fears the most is not fecal incontinence and urgency, but rather an attack of nausea and vomiting that would incapacitate him and leave him in desperate need of help, perhaps from unsympathetic strangers. But he is also anxious about the possibility of diarrhea and has been following a fairly strict low FODMAP diet for about two years.

Ever since the start of the COVID pandemic, he has been working primarily from home, which has been both a blessing and a curse. He feels safe and secure at home, so it is very easy for him when he's there, but he also realizes that his world is starting to get very small, and that he is getting increasingly anxious about even small trips to run errands or to go out to eat. His wife works as a surgical physician's assistant and is gone on long shifts four days a week. She is usually incredibly supportive, sympathetic, and understanding, but is starting to get frustrated with him about the way his limitations are impacting their life. They recently got a wedding invitation for a college friend of his who is getting married on the other side of the country, and he panicked when he thought about having to fly and travel around a new place. Given that he had been a confident and experienced world traveler earlier in his life, this made him realize that it was time to seek treatment. Nevertheless, he was quite relieved when the therapist agreed to see him via telehealth so he wouldn't have to travel to the therapist's office.

Session 1

The therapist starts the session by setting an agenda and letting Arun know that this is mostly a chance for them to get to know each other and for the therapist to hear his story, but that they will need to save some time at the end to teach him a very specific skill. The therapist asks Arun if he has ever been in therapy before, and what his expectations are about the process. He says he had a few sessions with a different therapist, but it didn't go very well. That therapist seemed most interested in hearing what his life was like growing up in India. He mostly felt like he was indulging their curiosity and it didn't feel very helpful at all. The therapist didn't really know anything about IBD, and he suspected they viewed him as an "exotic" oddity more than a person in need of specific help. The therapist thanks him for sharing that, and apologizes on behalf of the profession for his unfortunate experience. The therapist also assures him that CBT is indeed very problem focused and collaborative and that they will do their best to help him with his specific concerns. The therapist also asks him to let them know if the therapy ever starts to feel unhelpful or uncomfortable. "I know that can be hard, and seems to put an extra burden on you, but I want to do my best to make sure I'm meeting your needs, and if you tell me when I've screwed up, I can do my utmost to own it and get us back on the right track." Arun thanks the therapist for broaching this issue, and says "Yeah, this already feels better than it did with the other therapist."

Note that some white therapists might be thinking to themselves something like "It is highly likely that the prior therapist was psychodynamically oriented and was just trying to get a full family of origin history. It may not have been about race or culture at all." I would caution a therapist from saying such a thing. Remember, it's about race if the person of color thinks it's about race, because it *is* about race for them. Whether or not the prior therapist had a different goal in mind entirely and didn't intend and probably wasn't even aware of the fact that their line of questioning might be making Arun feel "exoticized" is irrelevant. The fact is, it *did* make him feel that way. So it *was* about race.

The therapist then asks Arun to share the history of his GI issues, and what he is struggling with currently. The therapist is horrified to learn of the hospital acquired *C. diff* infection, and expresses sympathy and outrage that this happened to him. The therapist also acknowledges how common agoraphobia and health anxiety can be for someone in Arun's position. They validate the ease and comfort of working from home, and praise him for recognizing that it was time to start pushing back against his anxiety. The therapist also gathers a bit more information about his diet. Arun was raised in a vegetarian household and still follows a strict vegetarian diet. His wife is actually a vegan, and they used to really enjoy cooking both traditional Indian foods, like dals (lentil soups) and chole masala (chickpea curries) and modern vegan dishes, many of which were also based on legumes. Ever since he was told by his gastroenterologist to follow the Low FODMAP Diet, his diet has become extremely limited, and that is one of the things his wife is most frustrated about. He eats a lot of plain white rice and potatoes now, and a limited selection of green vegetables (like steamed spinach) and small servings of homemade tomato or coconut milk based simmer sauces with no garlic or onion. He still eats yogurt and eggs, which are his main source of protein, but since his wife doesn't, they often don't eat the same meal anymore. This feels like a real loss of intimacy and shared pleasure, and he wishes he could expand his diet. Together, they establish that his main goals for treatment are to reduce the anticipatory anxiety and avoidance he feels around traveling outside the home, and to expand his diet back to what he used to enjoy. The therapist then takes a few minutes to teach him deep diaphragmatic breathing. He has had a daily yoga and mindfulness meditation practice for many years, and this comes quite naturally to him. It had never occurred to him to use the DDB separately to try to address his anxiety or nausea and cramping, and he is pleased to learn about this "bio-hack" that will let him control his heart rate, blood pressure, and even digestion.

At the end of the session the therapist asks Arun how the hour had felt, and whether it seemed like they were on the right track to addressing his specific concerns. "Absolutely," he said. "This feels really problem focused, and I appreciate that you asked about what was important to me. I'm also a really practical, technical guy, and I love learning new skills. It's cool that breathing can make such a difference, and I will definitely practice that this week."

Session 2

Arun reports that he did indeed practice the DDB over the week and finds it quite helpful. However, he had an experience over the weekend that was very troubling. "My wife and I want to build a shelf for a weird corner in our apartment, and we planned to go to the home store to pick up the supplies. I was getting super anxious about it all morning, which I know is ridiculous, but I kept imagining myself getting really sick in the car or at the home store. We went out to the car and got in and drove about half a block and I started to feel really panicky. I tried deep breathing, but it didn't help. My wife offered to drive, but that almost feels worse. At least when I'm driving I'm in control and I can decide to turn around. In the end, I bailed. We got about five blocks from our place and I just turned around and drove home. I couldn't do it. My wife was really annoyed and frustrated, and honestly so was I. I feel totally pathetic, but I just couldn't face it. This can't go on. I'll have no life left!"

The therapist empathizes with his dilemma, and agrees that when you are truly panicky, deep breathing may not be enough. The therapist then explains the basic cognitive model of panic—how we can entertain catastrophic distortions about basically benign body sensations and situations, and how scary imagery can exacerbate the panic. They map out several different pathways to treat this, including imaginal rescripting (imagining more benign and realistic outcomes), imaginal exposure (imaging the worst outcome over and over until it feels boring and silly) and *in vivo* exposure therapy. Arun opts for a combination of imaginal rescripting and *in vivo* exposure therapy.

Together they proceed to do an imaginal rescripting exercise in session. The therapist has Arun imagine that he is driving and begins to feel some abdominal discomfort and nausea. Arun acknowledges that he would usually start to feel quite anxious in that situation. The therapist suggests that Arun imagine a "coping effectively" outcome in which he takes some deep breaths, the panic recedes, and he continues driving on to his destination, despite feeling slightly nauseated. They then imagine a scenario in which he is feeling so nauseous, he actually needs to pull over and stop driving for a time.

"Imagine sitting back, closing your eyes, and just breathing. As the panic and nausea recede, imagine opening your eyes, sitting up, and getting back on the road," the therapist coaches. For the final scenario, they imagine that he is so nauseated he needs to pull over, open the door, and vomit into the street. "That would be pretty awful" he says. But together they imagine him rinsing his mouth out with the water bottle he usually has in the car, wiping his mouth, and continuing on his way. "I usually do feel a lot better if I actually vomit," he concedes. "It was only during the *C. diff* that it didn't really help."

After this series of exercises, the therapist suggests that Arun practice making a number of short trips during the week. "Even if you don't have anywhere you need to go, just drive around town for ten minutes. Better yet, run to the market or the pharmacy to pick up a few things. Have a destination you need to reach. Just be sure you do something every day." Arun agrees to this homework and leaves the session determined to conquer his fears.

Session 3

Arun is making incremental progress with his *in vivo* exposure therapy. He did indeed manage to get out and drive every day, even if only for ten minutes. Once when his wife worked a particularly grueling ten hour shift he agreed to drive to the hospital to pick her up. "I got super anxious leading up to it," he said. "I'm still getting this ridiculous anticipatory anxiety. But I made myself get in the car and do it. I knew I couldn't bail because she was counting on me to pick her up. The anxiety went away for a while, but when I hit the halfway point between our apartment and her work—what I call the point of no return—it kicked in again. I felt super anxious until she was in the car and we were actually on the way home. Then it receded, and by the time we got home I felt fine."

Arun and the therapist discuss his fears further, in particular his worry about being "incapacitated" while driving. He admits that he's also a bit worried about being pulled over by the police. "I'm documented, and I'm not black, but I'm still a brown skinned immigrant," he says. "What if the police think I'm driving erratically? What if I need to pull over on the highway onto the shoulder and a state trooper pulls up behind me? You have no idea how scary it can be for someone like me. Any legal entanglement could screw up my visa or my green card application and basically ruin my life." The therapist acknowledges that, as a white citizen, they cannot fully understand the fear of the police that many brown skinned people live with every day, because it is simply not part of their lived experience. "Yeah, I know," says Arun. "There's no way you could truly get it. On the other hand, if I'm being honest with myself, I don't think that's what I'm really scared of in the moment. It's more this feeling of helplessness—like I'm going to be desperate and ill and won't be able to take care of myself and no one will help. Sometimes I picture myself just collapsed on the sidewalk covered in vomit and diarrhea with everyone just walking past either ignoring me or looking at me with disgust."

The therapist suggests some further imaginal rescripting during the session, and encourages Arun to continue practicing driving and going out and about. "There's a local arts festival in our neighborhood my wife really wants to go to this weekend. That actually feels kind of anxiety provoking. I guess I'll make myself go to that," Arun suggests. The therapist agrees that that sounds like a perfect homework assignment.

Session 4

Arun and his wife went to the arts festival, and he had an "okay" time. "The anxiety kept coming in waves," he reports. "I was anxious in the morning before we left, then calmed down on the walk there, and then got anxious all over again when I realized it was crowded. I kept telling myself I could just run home if I felt sick or needed to use the restroom, but then I also kept thinking that I shouldn't think that—isn't that kind of like avoidance?" The therapist agrees that constantly mapping out "escape" plans for himself might actually be part of the problem, but praises him for sticking it out at the festival. "In the end we bought a really nice piece by a local artist, and we picked up some food from our favorite vegan restaurant and ate it while we wandered around. I was kind of worried about the food, but I ate it anyway. I tried to order something low FODMAP friendly. I don't think I could have done any of that a month ago. But by the end I was really itching to get home and relax. I still don't like crowds and feeling trapped far away from a clean restroom with the amenities I'm used to."

The therapist asks what he means by "amenities" and he shares that every time he moves into a new apartment in the US, the first thing he does is to install a bidet attachment in the toilet. "You Americans and your toilet paper! I'm sorry, but it's so gross! You have to put your hand back there, the paper shreds and it never gets you really clean. Bidets work *way* better. That's what

I grew up with. My wife was skeptical at first, but now she hates using anything else." He notes that there are small portable "travel" bidet bottles, but that they can be a little awkward to fill with water in a public restroom, especially one with motion sensors on the sinks. The therapist shares that bidets are a new idea to them, but that it makes a lot of sense. Indeed, the therapist says they will consider installing one in their own bathroom, and will suggest it to other patients with IBD as well. The therapist notes that they typically recommend that patients purchase some of the flushable wet wipes for adults that are now available. "They come in convenient, discreet little travel packs, and they work far better than dry toilet paper. That might be a good compromise for you when you're out and about." Arun had not heard of these, and said he might give them a try.

Together they talk through the rest of the exposure assignments he engaged in over the week. It is getting easier to "make" himself do things, but he is still experiencing considerable anticipatory anxiety before each venture, and the anxiety continues to wax and wane throughout each assignment. He always feels better when he is "on the way home" and he is still very worried about the cross country flight and long wedding weekend that is coming up in a couple of months. He also deeply wants to travel home to India in the upcoming fall to see his family before he and his wife initiate the green card application. "I've got to get this under control," he says.

Session 5

Arun reports that he managed several bigger trips over the week, including a drive out to the suburbs to visit a large computer hardware supply store to get some things he needed for his home office. They also got to the home store to get the wood, nails, and stain for the shelf they intended to build. All in all he is cautiously optimistic about the progress he is making, but is still frustrated by the "irrational anxiety" he keeps experiencing. "I feel like I'm getting better at plowing ahead despite feeling anxious, and not just looking for any excuse to cancel or bail, but I'd *really* prefer to not feel so anxious to begin with. I can't figure out why I'm still so scared. It doesn't make any sense."

The therapist encourages Arun to "go deep" and try to identify what he is actually most scared of. Say they were driving and he did feel nauseous, even to the point of needing to stop the car and vomit on the sidewalk or run into a store to have diarrhea, or worst yet have to poop on the verge of the highway.

What would be so terrible about that? It would be inconvenient, a little gross, maybe embarrassing, but not actually dangerous. Arun considers this. "But what if I was really incapacitated? What if I needed help and no one could help me?" The therapist presses this point a bit further, wondering why and how that might happen. Arun struggles to explain why this fear feels so deep and real. Even when he was at his most sick with the *C. diff* infection, he *did* in fact get the help he needed. It was an awful experience, but he didn't actually feel that panicked at the time. He knew he was ill and that he was going to get help. The therapist finally asks him "Is there any *other* time in your life when you've felt that way?"

In an "aha" moment, Arun realizes that he had an experience in his youth that may well be contributing to this. His family enjoyed traveling and when he was 13 they visited Nepal. On a short three day trek into the mountains that was supposed to be easy and for beginners, with a top altitude of about 7000 feet, his father suddenly developed altitude sickness. Initially he just felt a headache and some nausea, but it soon progressed to vomiting, disorientation, shortness of breath, and lack of coordination. Arun remembers the experience being terrifying. Despite the fact that their guide spoke excellent English and some Hindi, he remembers feeling frantic about not knowing what was wrong with his father or whether he was going to die. He knew they were in a foreign country, far from the urban center of Delhi where they lived and knew all the good hospitals. His mother was screaming at the guide to get them down off the mountain, and he and his little sister kept trying to calm her down while also feeling panicked and bewildered themselves. In the end, his father was fine. They got him down to a lower elevation and the altitude sickness resolved relatively quickly. But the memory of that trip—the fear and helplessness, the terror of a sudden onset of illness and feeling like you were far away from help and safety—seems to be the underlying template for Arun's current anxiety. "Wow," he says. "I can't believe that's been under the surface this whole time. Crazy that it never occurred to me before that that experience might have something to do with this. I always just assumed it was something about my own illness."

The therapist praises Arun for identifying this memory, which sounds fairly traumatic, even though it had a good outcome, and notes that his own illness probably resonated with that memory so much, it dredged up the old fear without really attaching it explicitly to the biographical memory itself. The therapist has Arun tell the story several more times, first from his childhood perspective with all the fear and confusion he felt at the time, and then from an adult perspective, with a new understanding of what his father was actually experiencing, his mother's urgency, the competence of the guide who assisted them in getting his father down the mountain, to the local village and back to the city, and the excellent attention he received from a medic back in Kathmandu. "Interesting," Arun concedes. "The story feels really different when I tell it from an adult perspective. It's almost like I've been seeing the world through the eyes of that 13 year old kid who felt so scared and helpless, thinking that that's still me." The therapist praises Arun for confronting the trauma of that experience and agrees that he is now a competent adult who can take care of himself, or reach out appropriately to others if he is truly in trouble or needs help. The therapist encourages Arun to take this new insight back out into the world, and see how the exposure therapy goes moving forward.

Session 6

Arun reports with pleasure that the exposure therapy is now going much better. (This suggests that his "aha" moment in the previous session led to what is known technically as a sudden gain in progress in psychotherapy.) "I'm still getting a little anticipatory anxiety, but I just pat my 13 year old self on the head and assure him that 'I've got this' and he doesn't need to worry. It seems silly, but it really helps. I've had a few instances of feeling queasy or crampy when I was out on the road, but it's not making me panic the same way. Mostly I just roll my eyes and tell myself it will pass, and it almost always does. One time I kept feeling lightheaded and queasy and weird, and I finally realized I was just hungry. Which reminds me, I'd really like to talk about my diet again. I'm getting really sick of eating just rice and potatoes all the time. But I'm kind of scared to reintroduce all the high FODMAP foods. I don't want my proctitis to suddenly flare again."

The therapist agrees that they seem to have addressed his first goal for treatment, and that it is indeed time to turn their attention to his second goal of expanding his diet. First, the therapist asks if Arun has ever spoken to a knowledgeable dietician about IBD and the Low FODMAP Diet. It turns out that Arun's gastroenterologist simply gave him a one page handout with high FODMAP foods "to avoid" and that was it. The therapist takes the time to educate him about the nature of high FODMAP foods, the problem with following a low FODMAP diet long term, and the worrisome effects on the microbiome. Since he suffered from a *C. diff* infection, it is particularly important for him to expand his diet and start including a wide variety of pre-biotic foods again. The therapist also acknowledges the importance of traditional cuisine and sharing cooking and eating with his wife as major sources of joy and pleasure in his life. The therapist suggests Arun consider a consultation with a knowledgeable registered dietician, to which he replies "I don't know—you seem to know so much about this, can't I just work with you?" The therapists graciously thanks Arun for his confidence in their knowledge and expertise, and agrees to provide initial guidance, but reaffirms the recommendation that at least a one-time consult with a highly skilled registered dietician (RD) could be important, and provides Arun with the name of an RD they have collaborated with in the past.

In the meantime, the therapist suggests that Arun pick one or two things he misses the most and consider a trial of reintroducing those foods one at a time. They remind him that he is likely to experience some gas and intestinal discomfort, especially if he chooses to reintroduce legumes like lentils, chickpeas, or beans, and not to panic if that happens. The therapist suggests that Arun consider ordering an enzyme product that will help break down the various carbohydrates that tend to be the worst offenders when it comes to gas and fermentation. "We want to set you up for success with this," they note. Eventually his own microbiome should bounce back and be able to manage these foods with a minimum of discomfort, but the transition can be uncomfortable. Arun remembers that he had a brief stint in college when he decided to eat chicken and fish, and initially had trouble digesting them, but then his digestion "got used to those foods" and he was able to eat them without discomfort. "I never really got used to the idea of eating an animal's flesh though. It always bothered me. That's why it was so hard to be told I couldn't eat any legumes anymore." Arun plans to try a few spoonfuls of a mild dal several days in a row, since that is the dish he has missed the most. "It won't taste the same without garlic and onions and all the spices we normally use, but at least I'll feel like I'm getting proper protein again." The therapist agrees that this is a good plan.

Session 7

Arun reports some "mixed success" with the reintroduction of foods. He decided to try the (lentil) dal several nights in a row, and then on another night also had a chickpea dish prepared with a garam masala (a blend of Indian spices) based on his mother's special recipe. "Oh my ... it was *so* good. I've missed real food." The lentils sat well two days in a row, but the night after he ate the chickpeas he experienced terrible gas pain, gurgling, and bloating. The next morning he had explosive diarrhea. "Guess I overdid it on that one," he notes ruefully. The therapist urges him again to consider consulting with the dietician and to not give up hope of expanding his diet. He may just need to take things slowly. He is anxious about the possibility of exacerbating his proctitis. "It's been under really good control for a while now—I really don't want to go back to that burning pain, urgency, and mucus in my stool." The therapist once again urges him to schedule a consultation with a dietician, but encourages him to keep cautiously and judiciously reintroducing small amounts of his favorite foods, and to not panic when he has an initial bad reaction.

They now turn their attention to thinking through the upcoming wedding and cross country travel. The therapist has Arun walk through all the different parts of the trip that make him nervous, and together they do both planful problem solving and some imaginal exposure and rescripting. By the end of the session, Arun is still anxious about it, but is reasonably confident that he will be able to make the trip. "I really hope my diet is back to normal by then—the friend who's getting married is Indian and so is his fiancé. I'm sure the food will be fabulous at all the various events, and I don't want to miss out on it!"

At this point Arun mentions that he thinks he'd like to take a break from therapy, at least for a while. "I feel like you've helped me a lot, and I'm in a much better place now. I know I still have some challenges to overcome, and yes, I promise to set up the consultation with the dietician, but I feel like I have the insight and the tools now to figure this out on my own moving forward." The therapist is a bit surprised, but quickly pivots to reinforcing the progress Arun has made, and agrees that he is indeed in a much better place. The therapist then spends the last few minutes doing some relapse prevention work, reviewing the skills and the new perspective he has arrived at, and praising all the hard work he was willing to do around exposure therapy. They also raise the issue of thinking about needing to get more colonoscopies in the future, and wonder if Arun will be anxious about the prospect, given his terrible experience with the *C. diff* infection. "Well, I'll definitely have a long talk with my doctor about better infection control procedures and what, if anything, will be done differently. I'll also be sure to take some probiotics and eat a normal varied diet in the months leading up to it so my microbiome is in better shape. I'm sure I'll be super anxious about it when the time comes. But I know that infections are actually quite rare after routine colonoscopies. So I'll try to use all the things you taught me about not catastrophizing or imagining the worst outcomes or at least imagine myself coping effectively if something does go wrong. You really have given me new tools to manage all this and I'm very grateful." The therapist smiles warmly and says "I'm glad to know this felt helpful, but I also want *you* to take credit for all the hard work you did! Doing exposure therapy takes courage and determination, and you did it—almost every day!" The therapist assures Arun that if he ever feels like he needs a quick booster session, they are happy to be available.

Two months later the therapist got a text message from Arun with several photos of himself and his wife at the wedding, dancing, celebrating, and *eating*. "I couldn't have done it without you!" his message said. "Thanks for everything."

Case 5–Sandy

Sandy is a 57 year old, white, cis-gendered, straight, once divorced, once widowed woman. She lives in a fairly rural community and has to drive over an hour to see her doctor. She has had a truly traumatic and difficult life, filled with medical crises and loss. She has severe Crohn's disease that is not under good medical control. She suffers from strictures, has several fistulas, including a rectal–vaginal fistula, and has had several resection surgeries, including a time with an ostomy. Both of her biological children also had or have Crohn's disease. Her daughter died ten years ago of a fentanyl overdose at age 28, after developing an opiate dependence on painkillers prescribed by her doctor to manage pain secondary to Crohn's disease. Her son is suffering from progressive Crohn's as well. He is in the military, and refused biologic medication for years because it renders a service member non-deployable, and would have dramatically curtailed his career opportunities. He now also has stricturing disease, and copes with frequent transient small bowel obstructions that lead to vomiting and pain. Sandy and her first husband divorced acrimoniously when she was 29, and her children were eight and ten. She remarried several years later to a man she described as "the love of my life." Tragically, he died about seven years later in a construction accident when he fell off the second story of a home he was building. Sandy supports herself with piecemeal, mostly remote work as a bookkeeper for several local businesses. She depends on Medicaid for health insurance, and cannot afford private pay therapy

Sandy smokes, which is now precluding surgical correction of her fistula. Her surgeon told her "It won't heal if you keep smoking. I'm not going to waste my time repairing something that's just going to tear open again. If you're going to keep smoking, you might as well shoot yourself." Needless to say, she experienced this comment as fairly hurtful, and it did not motivate her to quit smoking. Sandy is severely depressed, anxious, and in pain much of the time. She is lonely and isolated. She is also overweight, but undernourished. She has some medical comorbidities as well—she is pre-diabetic, and has some mild congestive heart failure, with chronic swelling in her legs and ankles. The good news is that she doesn't drink alcohol or use opiates herself. Nevertheless, she comes to therapy with a host of problems that might seem insurmountable at first glance. The therapist does not accept Medicaid, but has a number of full fee clients in their practice, so agrees to see Sandy *pro bono* for a nominal fee of $10 per session.

Session 1

As always, the therapist begins the session by taking a thorough history. As Sandy's story unfolds, it seems there is a new trauma at every turning. Even the therapist starts to feel overwhelmed by the degree of loss Sandy has experienced. Sandy weeps a good deal during the session, castigating herself for many perceived flaws. She refers to her deceased daughter as "my angel in heaven" and blames herself for not somehow saving her from opiate addiction. The therapist takes the opportunity to empathize with her loss—agreeing that losing a child is probably the worst pain there is—but then gently guides Sandy to consider that many IBD patients developed opiate addictions when treated (inappropriately but all too commonly) with narcotic painkillers for poorly managed IBD. Sandy admits that her own doctor also recommended opiates at one point. "I guess I got lucky—they made me feel kind of nauseous and they really constipated me, so I got off them right away. My angel girl wasn't so lucky."

Sandy's first husband, Mike, was distant and emotionally abusive. They married when she was 18 and he was 24, because she was pregnant with their daughter, who was born just after Sandy turned 19. "He always told me I was lazy and looking for any excuse to not do the housework or cook for him. He didn't get how sick I was sometimes, or how cooking things I couldn't eat was no fun. He didn't even drive me to any of my doctor's appointments. When I had my first colonoscopy, I had to ask my sister to go with me. It's embarrassing thinking back on it. I don't know why I stayed with him as long as I did. If it hadn't been for the babies, I would have left his ass a lot faster." Her second husband, Tom, was kind and caring. "He was the love of my life. He didn't care about my scars or needing to rest up sometimes or go to the bathroom a lot. He was a simple guy—didn't need much. He was just happy to see me when he got home. He'd help with dinner and dishes. He was a real good step dad too, and a good daddy to his little girl with his ex. The kids loved him, especially my son. He taught him all about tools and building things and fixing the car. Other than my angel baby dying, his accident was the worst thing that ever happened to me—and that's saying something. If it hadn't been for the kids, I think my will to live would have died with him. My son decided to sign up right after he died. He was only 17. I had to sign a waiver for him and everything. So then I kind of lost him too."

The therapist empathizes with all the loss Sandy has experienced, and praises her for her resilience in the face of so much loss and trauma. "I guess

I never saw it that way," Sandy says. "I just figured you had to keep going." The therapist agrees that one does indeed "have to keep going" but points out that Sandy managed to keep her family together, earn enough to pay the mortgage and put food on the table, and managed to keep body and soul together for herself and her children. "Huh," Sandy says. "I kind of see myself as pathetic. But I guess maybe you have a point."

The therapist then goes on to ask more about Sandy's IBD. They are horrified to hear what the surgeon told her. "I'm so sorry the doctor said that to you—that's horrible," the therapist says. "Oh, that's not unusual," Sandy replies. "When you're overweight and you smoke you get used to doctors saying stuff like that. Every doctor I see makes some snide remark about how I'm basically choosing to kill myself and I should just act different and make better choices. Humph. As if it were that easy." The therapist expresses their sympathy for Sandy being on the receiving end of so much bias and so many ham-handed attempts to intervene by people in the medical community. She then asks Sandy what *her* goals are for treatment.

"Well I don't really know. I signed up for this because I saw a flyer at the doctor's office, but I guess I don't really know what you can do to help. Feels sort of good to talk about stuff though, even though it also kinda hurts." The therapist replies that they're glad it feels good to talk about things, but they also want to be sure that they are helping Sandy make positive changes in her life that *she* actually wants to make.

Sandy admits that the rectal–vaginal fistula is probably the thing that is bothering her the most. "It's super embarrassing. I'm sure I stink all the time. I keep getting infections. I have to wash all the time. I wear Depend's diapers even when I'm at home. I don't go out much or see people because of it. I would really love to be able to get that fixed." The therapist agrees that that seems like a good long term goal, and asks Sandy what is getting in the way. "Well, I gotta quit smoking for one thing. I also wonder if I should try one of these medications my doctor is always pushing me to take. I've used a lot of steroids in my life. My doctor always wants me to try something new, but I'm nervous about all the side effects with those drugs. Crohn's is bad enough—I bet you anything with my luck, I'm the one who gets cancer if I try something else."

The therapist reflects back to Sandy that it sounds like quitting smoking and perhaps thinking about trying a new Crohn's medication would allow her to get the fistula corrected (or might even allow it to heal on its own) and that that would go a long way toward improving her quality of life. "Yeah,

I could start going out again, seeing my friends. Visit my sister. My step daughter Stephanie is a real sweet girl and she has a little baby herself now. I'd love to babysit for her when I can." The therapist then asks Sandy what the hardest thing about quitting smoking would be. "Well I just get so nervous and crabby when I try to quit. I can't stand the cravings. I get crazy hungry every time I've tried, and I'm already too fat. It's like a good friend, you know? Always there, reliable, makes you feel good. Kind of like Tom was." The therapist agrees that nicotine does indeed have a number of powerful positive effects, including working as both an anxiolytic *and* a cognitive stimulant, and empathizes with how difficult it is to quit. However, they point out that a good friend doesn't try to kill you. "Cigarettes are a pretty treacherous friend, aren't they?" They then suggest getting nicotine patches and gum to help with the cravings. They also segue to teaching deep breathing. "It's not as powerful as nicotine," the therapist acknowledges. "But deep breathing can help take the edge off of feeling anxious and irritable." Sandy struggles a bit to master the deep breathing and actually starts coughing at one point during the exercise. But she keeps trying and manages to take a few calming deep breaths. Her homework is to go to Walmart to buy some nicotine patches and gum and to practice deep breathing.

Session 2

Sandy returns for the second session feeling irritable and somewhat out of sorts. She reports that she did try to buy the nicotine patches, but was overwhelmed by how expensive they were. She decided she couldn't possibly afford them, which was incredibly frustrating. She bought a single pack of Nicorette gum, and tried to use it to replace a few cigarettes, but found that it burned her mouth and made her feel somewhat nauseous, so she gave up on it. The therapist apologizes for not having thought about the cost, and spends a few minutes in session looking up Medicaid coverage of tobacco-dependence treatments. It turns out that in their state (indeed in almost all states) Medicaid will cover the entire expense of nicotine patches. Sandy is surprised and relieved to hear this. "Oh, okay," she says. "I guess I'll go back to the store and get them after all." The therapist assures Sandy that the smoking cessation literature suggests that quitting is much more likely to be successful if you use a nicotine replacement product, and that it should dramatically reduce her cravings and withdrawal symptoms.

The therapist now requests Sandy's permission to speak to her gastroenter-ologist. The therapist wants to understand her current treatment regimen and which medication the GI doc would like Sandy to start. Sandy agrees and gives her the doctor's contact information. The therapist also has Sandy sign a bi-directional release of information, since it would be difficult for Sandy to stop in to the doctor to sign one there. Sandy notes that she has been on and off prednisone "more times than I can count. Of course, I *always* get the damn moon face and look even fatter than I am. But it does help. I don't really under-stand why my doctor won't just let me stay on it. I always feel better when I'm taking it." The therapist takes this opportunity to do some psychoeducation with Sandy about the risks of staying on steroids long term. "My momma broke her hip when she was 73," Sandy confides. "She never walked right after that. I guess getting osteoporosis would be bad, huh?" The therapist agrees with this, and asks Sandy what she remembers about what the doctor has recommended. "I think he said something about going to an infusion center. It was for remi … something. Remillera? Rumira? I'm not sure. He said I'd have to get a bunch of infusions at first, and then go back for them every six to eight weeks. Or maybe he said I could maybe give myself shots. I don't know if I could do that. It seems like a big commitment. A lot of time driving and sitting around not working." It is clear from this narrative that Sandy does not remember which medication her GI doc actually recommended, and is confusing the names of several that might have been presented to her as options, including Remicade, Stelara, and Humira. Sandy clearly needs help interpreting and understanding her doctor's recommendations. Nevertheless, the therapist should take seriously Sandy's concerns about taking time out of work. She is paid hourly or by the job, and every day she has to take off to go get treatment is a day's earnings she doesn't make.

The therapist takes some time to discuss Sandy's other concerns about medication, and encourages her to think about the risks of *not* taking the medicine. Sandy is afraid of cancer, but the therapist points out that poorly managed Crohn's dramatically increases the risk of cancer as well. "I guess I never thought about it that way," Sandy admits. They also take a few minutes to look up where the closest infusion center is to where she lives. It turns out the general hospital several towns over has one. "I looked those up before, but I thought those were just for cancer patients," Sandy says. The therapist acknowledges that most infusion centers treat both cancer and GI patients, and that their names often have "Cancer Center" in the title, which could be confusing. "Of course, we will need to make sure that your GI doc is affiliated with that center and can actually send you there, but I bet it would be doable. And if you choose one of the medications that you can give yourself by injection, you wouldn't even have to take time off work. I'm sure you can learn to do it. They have nurses to teach you. These medicines really are far more effective than steroids. I think you should go for it." Sandy admits that perhaps it wouldn't be as overwhelming as she thought to start a new medication, and agrees to consider it after the therapist talks to her GI doc.

The rest of the session is spent discussing Sandy's grief over her daughter's death. She describes the two years leading up to it, the midnight phone calls, multiple crises and attempts to rescue her daughter. She describes the day two police officers showed up at her door. She assumed her daughter had been arrested for possession, but they informed her that her daughter had died. She remembers standing there just rooted to the floor in shock. "I don't think anything even came out of my mouth. I just stared at them. I think they said something about where to go to ID her body, but I just felt numb all over and could barely hear them. I did eventually get to the morgue. That was the hardest thing I ever had to do in my whole life. When they pulled that sheet back and I saw my angel baby lying there all cold and pale, I just started wailing. Honestly that moment haunts me every day and every night. More so than the day I found out Tom had died. That was bad, for sure, but this—well nothing compares. I wouldn't wish that pain on my worst enemy. And it never goes away."

The therapist empathizes with the horror of this trauma, and asks Sandy some gentle, but thorough questions about the symptoms of PTSD. Sandy falls just one symptom short of meeting criteria, but it is clear to the therapist that Sandy would benefit from a course of trauma specific therapy. She tells Sandy that there are things they can do together that might make the pain easier to bear, and describes several approaches to trauma work they could try. Sandy is skeptical, but likes the idea of imaginal rescripting and agrees to give it a try.

Sandy's homework that week is to try again to pick up nicotine patches from Walmart (which should be free with Medicaid) and to call her doctor to set up an appointment to discuss trying a new medication.

After Sandy leaves, the therapist places a call to Sandy's GI doctor, pressing "1" for "If this is a physician or doctor's office calling." Amazingly, his nurse assistant is able to grab him out of office hours and he comes to the phone right away. "I have been trying *for years* to get that woman onto an appropriate biologic immunosuppressive medication!" he says with some exasperation.

"I've explained all about the risks and offered her Humira, Remicade, and even Stelara. She only ever agrees to prednisone, despite the severity of her disease. It's incredibly frustrating. I don't know what magic you worked, but if she's finally willing to start a TNF or IL inhibitor that would be fantastic. I'll have our scheduler reach out to her to set her up." The doctor is not affiliated with the closest infusion center, but is affiliated with one just 15 minutes further away.

Session 3

Session three starts out with a review of the therapist's conversation with the GI doc. Sandy confirms that his office reached out to her. He wants her to come in for an in person appointment to discuss the different options. She asked him to *please* make it a telehealth visit so she didn't have to spend so much time driving, and he agreed. She has the appointment scheduled later in the week, and is reluctantly making her peace with the need for more aggressive treatment. "I guess you think I've been pretty dumb, huh? I know the doctor has always been annoyed with me. He doesn't get why I opted for surgery over medication. I don't know. All those medicines scare me more than surgery did. But I guess it's time to admit I have to try them. Cause he said he won't give me prednisone anymore until I do." The therapist assures Sandy that they don't think she's "dumb" for having concerns about side effects. But they also praise her for being open to new ways of thinking and for being brave enough to try a new medicine. They also express optimism that the new medication regimen will help her heal.

They now turn their attention to smoking cessation. Sandy was indeed able to purchase the patches, but has been too nervous to try them. The therapist explains the concepts of conditioned withdrawal and stimulus control and encourages Sandy to change up her routine around the times she usually lights up. The therapist also helps Sandy figure out what dose of patch to use, and walks her through a standard protocol. They even chart it out for a month to help Sandy keep track. Sandy then spontaneously pulls her pack of cigarettes out and holds it up in front of the camera. "Cigs—you are a bad friend. You pretend to like me and make me feel better, but you're actually killing me and making my life hell. If I don't quit you, I'll never get my life back. My body will never heal and I'll always smell like shit. So f*** you. We're done." She then dramatically crumples up the pack and tosses it over her shoulder. The therapist praises Sandy for this change of heart and commitment to smoking cessation, and reminds her that it will be hard, but that they have full confidence in her.

The therapist now has a decision to make. They could proceed with trauma work over the death of her daughter, or they could continue to evaluate her diet, nutritional status, social support, and other factors affecting resilience and quality of life. Unsure which way to proceed, the therapist asks Sandy what she would prefer. "I don't know if I can face the trauma stuff today," Sandy says. "I'm not chickening out or anything, but maybe we should talk about food. I'm real scared I'm going to gain even more weight now that I'm quitting." The therapist agrees to save the trauma work for another day, and proceeds to evaluate Sandy's diet.

It turns out that Sandy eats a very bland diet full of highly processed, "easy to digest" carbs. "I love saltines and pasta and macaroni and cheese." She says. "I'll eat cookies and toast and cereal. I like Honey Nut Cheerios and Cinnamon Toast Crunch. Sometimes I'll have an egg or a slice of American cheese. But I can't eat greens or too much fruit—they give me real bad gas and diarrhea, and I have a real hard time digesting things like chicken and pork. And *don't* ask me to eat fish. Smells like cat food. Gross. I can do a hamburger sometimes, and I like mashed potatoes. I try to avoid too much fried food, so I don't do fries. Honestly, I don't eat that much, and sometimes I only eat a few snacks and then dinner. I don't understand why I'm so heavy."

The therapist acknowledges that all of these foods are comforting and quite low in fiber, and thus "easy" to digest. But they point out that Sandy's diet is missing lots of important nutrients. It's fairly low in protein and has almost no fiber. It's missing a range of vitamins and minerals, and is a far cry from the healthy diet she needs to thrive. It's also filled with "carbs" which spike blood sugar. Sandy admits that her family doctor told her she is pre-diabetic. She had no idea that eating crackers and cereal could contribute to blood sugar spikes. They spend a good deal of the rest of the session educating Sandy about basic nutrition and coming up with various ideas for how she could try to expand her diet. The therapist asks Sandy if there are any vegetables that don't give her gas that she would be willing to try. "Well, I kinda like sweet potatoes and squash and maybe cooked carrots. Do they count? They may not be green, but at least they're orange!" The therapist notes that those are all fairly sweet, but that it would be a great way to start adding some variety back into her diet. She also suggests trying some berries, but Sandy shuts this down by saying "I can't afford them except in summer when I can go to a pick it yourself place. They're too expensive out of season." The therapist apologizes for overlooking this, but suggests the option of buying some frozen berries and putting them in a smoothie with some vanilla yogurt. "That might be good," Sandy acknowledges. For her homework, in addition to keeping the appointment with her doctor, she agrees to try adding a few new foods into her diet.

Session 4

Sandy kept the teletherapy appointment with her GI doctor and has reluctantly agreed to start a trial of Humira. "He said that's the one Medicaid will approve, and I don't have to go to the infusion center all the time. His nurse can show me how to do the injections the first time, and then I can just do it myself at home." He also wanted her to get blood work and a new fecal calprotectin test so they would have a baseline assessment of her level of inflammation at the beginning of treatment. She got the blood work done right away, and it turns out she is severely anemic and B12 and vitamin D deficient. He wants her to get an iron infusion and a B12 injection and start taking oral supplements. "This feels kinda like a rollercoaster now—I got on and I can't get off!" Sandy says sardonically. The therapist praises Sandy for forging ahead with all these aspects of her care so efficiently, and assures her that she should start feeling better in all sorts of ways as she puts these things in place. "Kinda ironic that I'm doing the Humira shots, but I still have to go to an infusion center to get the iron," Sandy quips.

Sandy has tried to increase the variety in her diet with some success, but her understanding of basic nutrition remains somewhat limited. "I found my memaw's recipe for sweet potato pie and made it. Damn it was good. I ate almost the whole thing, but I saved a few pieces for my step daughter and her husband. They came over last weekend to visit and I got to see the baby. That was nice." The therapist expresses pleasure for Sandy that she had a visit from her family, and praises her trying to expand her diet, but suggests a baked sweet potato or roasted squash would be a better choice, especially for someone who is pre-diabetic. "Yeah," says Sandy sheepishly. "I knew you would say that. I did try a ground turkey hash with a little shredded zucchini in it. It was okay I guess. Kinda watery and tasteless, but it didn't upset my stomach at all, so I guess that was a win." The therapist suggests a few different recipes Sandy could try that might be tastier and still healthful. Sandy expresses interest in learning new dishes, and asks the therapist to write some down for her.

On the good news front, she reports that she has not smoked a single cigarette all week. "That's the first time in 40 years I've been able to go that long," she says proudly. "These patches are pretty amazing. I miss the flavor and the ritual—you know, lighting up while I watch the morning shows or when I watch my shows at night. But I'm not *craving* it the way I always did when I tried to quit before. And I don't feel so miserable and crabby either. My sister is amazed. She said she might try to quit too. That'd be good, cause I don't think I can be around someone who's smoking without wanting one. My step daughter never smoked, bless her. Tom was a real good influence on her. She never did like it when I smoked at her house, even if I went outside. She's real proud of me for quitting—says she can bring the baby over more often now. So I guess even if I can't get this damn fistula fixed, quitting smoking is gonna be a good thing." The therapist celebrates these successes and points out that healthful behavior change can ripple outward in all kinds of good ways, helping other people make healthier choices and opening up new opportunities for social support.

Sandy then got quiet and tearful. "I just wish my angel girl had had a chance to quit those drugs. Maybe if I'd gotten help like this earlier, I would have been able to help her too before it was too late." The therapist acknowledges Sandy's perception of missed opportunities, but reminds her that opiate addiction is one of the very hardest things to beat. The therapist agrees, however, that if her daughter had gotten better care—like access to treatment with Suboxone—she might have stood a better chance. "It makes me so *MAD!*" Sandy wails. "My beautiful, sweet angel baby. I couldn't ever get anyone to help her. They just blamed her for being a drug addict. It wasn't her *FAULT!*" The therapist validates Sandy's rage and grief and gently suggests that it might be time to do some trauma work. Sandy agrees, but says "I'm so spittin' mad right now I'm not sure what you can do with me."

The therapist starts by encouraging Sandy to simply share her memories of her daughter—starting in her childhood and going all the way up to her death. Sandy takes a deep breath, and fills the rest of the session with lovely, heartwarming stories of her daughter's childhood, then the difficulty with getting her diagnosed with Crohn's. "Her teachers kept telling me I should just ignore her bellyaching and make her go to school. They thought she was faking it to stay home. But I knew better. My angel baby loved school. She would be crying curled up on her bedroom floor telling me her tummy hurt.

I kept going to different doctors till I finally got one that did the right tests. Mike was no help. He thought she was just bellyaching too." The therapist takes a moment to praise Sandy for her parental instincts and persistence in getting her daughter appropriately diagnosed. "Yeah, didn't really help in the end, though, did it. They diagnosed her alright, but then they started her on those damn pain pills." Sandy then tells the story of her daughter's descent into opiate dependence. "When the doctor started trying to wean her off, it was already too late. She started buying heroin off the street to manage the pain and the cravings I guess. And then some dealer sold her shit laced with fentanyl. And she died."

The therapist encourages Sandy to do some trauma writing as homework, including writing angry letters to the doctors who managed her daughter's care, to the ER docs and drug counselors who refused to give her Suboxone, and to the drug dealer who sold her the fatal dose.

Session 5

Sandy did write the letters and said it felt incredibly hard at first, but once she got going she just wrote and wrote and wrote. She cried while doing it, but in the end it felt quite cathartic. However, she is still tortured by the memory of seeing her daughter's body in the morgue. The therapist suggests a round of imaginal rescripting to work on that memory, and Sandy agrees. The therapist has Sandy close her eyes and begin with paced, mindful breathing. They then have Sandy imagine she is on the beach, using all five senses to construct a realistic, immersive environment. As she imagines walking down the beach, the therapist instructs her to imagine the front door of the morgue magically appearing in front of her. She has Sandy walk into the morgue and pause at the entrance, feeling the dread, noticing the flickering fluorescent lights and the horrible gray linoleum. Then she walks into the morgue room itself. Again, she needs to pause and remember the smells, the cold air, and the silence. She imagines the attendant walking to a vault in the wall and opening it up and sliding the gurney out. She sees the attendant pull back the sheet and allows herself to feel the shock and despair of seeing her daughter lying cold and still and dead. The therapist can see that Sandy is still, with her eyes closed, but tears are streaming down her cheeks. The therapist then talks Sandy through a rescripting. They narrate an image of Sandy's daughter starting to glow with a heavenly golden light. Then her spirit—glowing, perfectly beautiful, whole, and looking like herself at her healthiest, rises up out of the cold still body and gets up off the table. The spirit smiles at her mother warmly and reaches out to touch Sandy's hand, which tingles and glows. "I'm okay Mom," the spirit says. "Dying didn't hurt at all, and I truly am in a better place now. I'm sorry I can't be with you, but I don't want you to worry about me. I'm not in pain. I'm not struggling. I miss you, but I'll see you again someday. None of this is your fault. You were the best mom I could have asked for. You need to let me go now. Remember me like this—this is who I always was and still am." The therapist then has Sandy imagine the entire room dissolving in warm golden light until the morgue disappears and she finds herself back on the beach in the warm sunlight. The therapist allows Sandy to sit still and return her focus to the waves and the light sparkling on the water, then gently tells her to open her eyes whenever she is ready.

When Sandy opens her eyes, the therapist asks "How was that?" Sandy pauses to collect her thoughts, and wipes the tears off her face. "Wild. That was crazy," she says. "It seemed so real. I know it didn't really happen, but it feels like truth somehow. I always believed my baby girl was an angel in heaven. Now I know it in my bones. I think maybe I can just see the angel from now on, not the body." The therapist is pleased and tells Sandy that she hopes this exercise will help bring her peace moving forward. (For therapists who are unfamiliar with the power of imaginal rescripting, you should know that the mechanism of action is almost certainly based on the reconsolidation of the trauma memory with new emotional associations.)

They spend the remainder of the session touching base about Sandy's progress with smoking cessation (two weeks of abstinence thus far, though she was very tempted to beg a cigarette off a friend she met for coffee one day) and with expanding her diet. She has tried some smoothies, and even bought a bag of frozen mixed berries and kale to put in them. She also made a loaf of zucchini bread which she says "wasn't half bad." She is feeling better after the iron infusion and the B12 injection. She is also scheduled for her onboarding with Humira later in the week. She is very anxious about it, which the therapist helps her address. All in all, her energy is up a bit, and she is feeling more motivated and hopeful, although she is still struggling with chronic burning abdominal pain, watery diarrhea and what she calls "indigestion."

Her homework for the week is to get to her Humira onboarding appointment, and to continue with her plan for slowly decreasing the nicotine dose of the patches.

Session 6

Sandy reports that she had her training session with a nurse and it went "okay." "I'm still kind of freaked out about giving myself the shots, but I guess I'll get used to it. The bad news is I've gained five pounds. I knew that would happen if I tried to quit smoking." I was so stressed out about it all I bought a pack from a convenience store around the corner from the hospital and smoked three cigs in a row. Stupid. I forgot I had a patch on and I ended up feeling so jazzed and nauseous I could barely drive home. You'll be pleased to know I threw the rest away. Waste of damn money, the whole thing. At least the patches are free."

The therapist empathizes with Sandy's stress about starting Humira and acknowledges that setbacks during quitting are incredibly common and nothing to feel bad about. They also praise Sandy for throwing the rest of the pack away. The therapist then suggests that Sandy think about something she would like to buy for herself—something she normally wouldn't be able to afford, but could use the money she is saving on cigarettes to get for herself. "I have always wanted to get one of those fancy hot stone massages," Sandy says. "I'd feel real rich having someone pamper me that way. You know, ever since Tom died, I don't think I've been touched by anyone, except my step daughter's little baby. That's a long dry spell, you know? I don't think I'll ever date again. Who would want me? But just having someone lay their hands on me would feel awful nice." The therapist agrees that saving up for a massage is a terrific idea, and agrees that physical touch is an important part of well-being.

The therapist then turns their attention to the topic of physical activity. Sandy has been overweight, pre-diabetic, and malnourished for several years. She feels ugly—even disgusting—and hates her body. The therapist gently asks Sandy whether she has ever enjoyed any kind of physical activity. "Not really," Sandy says. "When my kids were little I didn't mind running around after them at the playground, but I've never been sporty or athletic. I hated gym. My son was a real talented athlete. The military was a good fit for him. But I never could do all that stuff—running and team sports. I was the girl who always kind of hid in the back of the gym or told the gym teacher I had my period so I could just go to the nurses' office." The therapist realizes that getting Sandy on board with a program of physical activity is going to be challenging, but persists, since exercise has so many benefits. They work on addressing Sandy's beliefs about exercise (it's embarrassing, it's uncomfortable, you have to be "good" at sports) and reframing the nature of physical activity. "I'm *never* going to go to a gym," Sandy states. "That's fine," replies the therapist. "I hate gyms too!"

Gently the therapist guides Sandy to consider what sort of physical activity she *might* enjoy. "Well you know, I always loved the idea of getting myself a little dog and taking it for walks around the neighborhood. I've just been so busy in my life, or in crisis or too sick to commit to it." The therapist is enthusiastic about this idea. "You know," they say, "another advantage of getting a dog is that it would snuggle with you. Dogs are a wonderful source of touch and physical affection. There's a lot of research showing that they help with depression and loneliness and even heart disease!" Together they spend a little time pulling up the local shelter's website to see what dogs might be available. Before she knows it, Sandy has fallen in love with a dog on the website, a five year old, handsome, 35 pound black and white neutered male described on the site as a "cuddle bug who loves nothing more than hanging out on the couch getting tummy rubs, but will happily go for walks with you too." "As long as he's good with the baby, he seems like he'd be perfect! He kind of reminds me of Tom a little. Tom had real dark hair and was handsome just like this guy." Sandy says. The therapist cautions Sandy about jumping in too quickly, but agrees that she should go ahead and set an appointment to meet the dog. They also suggest that Sandy read some basic dog training books to prepare herself for what owning a dog would truly be like.

The balance of the session is spent on reviewing her smoking cessation plan and thinking about meals and recipes she could try out.

Session 7

Sandy had sent the therapist a text message with a picture of her and her new dog, rechristened Tommy, from the shelter the day she adopted him, so the therapist is prepared when Sandy announces that "Tommy is the best thing that's happened to me in years!" She notes that having the dog in her life has motivated her to continue on this new path to health. "Tommy needs me! I have to take care of myself now." She reports that her step daughter was a little nervous about him, but agreed to bring the baby over. "Tommy was a good boy. He just licked the baby's face and made him giggle. Stephanie said she feels comfortable with him being around the baby, and she's glad to let me babysit." The therapist points out that there is considerable literature showing that exposure to pet cats and dogs early in life actually protects children from developing autoimmune disorders, like asthma, food allergies, and even IBD. "Well see, there you go!" Sandy adds. "My Tommy is a good boy and he's good for all of us!"

Sandy is due to give herself her second loading dose of Humira later in the week, and she and the therapist talk about some of her anxieties around injecting herself. The therapist suggests several resources, including YouTube videos posted by other patients with IBD demonstrating how to do it, and the Crohn's and Colitis Foundation peer to peer helpline. Sandy considers both of these and says she might do one of them. "I tried to find a CCF support group years ago but there were none near me, so I just gave up." The therapist points out that many of the support groups have moved online since the pandemic, so distance is much less of an issue now. "It would be nice to have people to talk to who get it," Sandy admits. "Besides you, I mean," she hastily adds. The therapist laughs and says of *course* Sandy should find support in her community. "MY job is to give you skills and help you through the stuck place you were in. But having ongoing support from others in the IBD community is a great idea."

The remainder of the session is spent on Sandy discussing the challenges of remaining smoke-free and trying to manage her diet and calorie intake. She speaks warmly about her step daughter Stephanie and how she feels like she's getting closer to that little family and how much it means to her. She also mentions that her son is going to be home on a short leave, and she can't wait to talk to him about the importance of pursuing treatment and not letting things get out of control. "I know he might feel like he's compromising his career, but one of the things you've helped me realize is that Crohn's can really mess up your whole life and just destroy your body if you don't get it treated. Whatever the downsides of treatment are, Crohn's is worse. I want him and me to thrive. I know we have our own angel girl in heaven looking out for us, and I know she'd want us to get good care." Sandy decides to skip a week of therapy in order to have time with her son.

Session 8

Sandy reports that she had a wonderful visit with her son, John. The two of them had some tough conversations about getting treatment, and he has agreed that the Crohn's itself is compromising his physical fitness and battle readiness so much that he really has no choice. He loved the new dog and the two of them went on some walks together with Tommy. He taught her a lot about dog training. "John and Tommy are both so smart, and John knows all about discipline. He had him heeling on leash lickety-split. I don't know if I'll be that good at it, but it showed me what Tommy is capable of."

She even made dinner for John and Stephanie's family. "I tried to include some veggies and some fiber and protein. We had my new zucchini spice bread for dessert. They couldn't believe it had vegetables in it! Even Stephanie's husband liked it, and he always says he's 'allergic' to 'green' things! Also, I lost two pounds this week. I guess walking Tommy is helping. The damn fistula makes it kind of uncomfortable, but that just makes me more determined than ever to quit smoking for good."

She reports that while the patches are helping (and she has adjusted the dose down a bit as planned) she still misses cigarettes terribly. "It's everything about them—the taste, the smoke, the ritual. It's been part of my life for so long I don't really know who I am without them. Sometimes I'll catch a whiff of someone's smoke and my whole body will just lean into it. Makes me long to light up myself." The therapist praises her for sticking with the smoking cessation plan, and reminds her that her primary goal was to get the fistula to either heal or to have it surgically corrected, and that quitting smoking is an essential part of achieving that. The therapist points out that people tend to think of themselves as "smokers, ex-smokers or non-smokers." They encourage Sandy to begin the shift to identifying first as an "ex-smoker" (rather than a smoker who is trying to quit) and then eventually to just think of herself as a "non-smoker."

They then spend some time reviewing where Sandy was when she started treatment, and what her primary goals were. Sandy is amazed to realize how much progress she has made. She reports almost as a side note that she successfully gave herself her second loading dose of Humira, and is due for the third dose in a few days. "It really wasn't that big a deal. I just needed to get over myself. Honestly, I am feeling a bit better already. I have a little less burning pain and the urgency is going down a bit. I'm really hoping the fistula may start to heal on its own and I never have to see that surgeon again." The therapist joins Sandy in hoping for such a good outcome.

They then spend some time reviewing what Sandy would still like to accomplish, and whether she would like to continue in therapy or wrap things up. "Well I don't want to lose you," Sandy confides. "You've helped me so much. I'm not sure I can keep doing all this on my own without your support. But I know you're seeing me basically for free and I feel kinda bad about that. I wish I could pay you what you deserve." The therapist assures Sandy that they are happy to keep working with her, but that it might be time to switch to every other week. Sandy agrees that this makes sense, and thanks the therapist for being both generous and flexible.

Sessions 9 and Beyond

Like Julie, Sandy is someone who will need ongoing support, guidance, advocacy and psychotherapy to make the most of her recovery. Although she made remarkable progress in a mere eight sessions, especially given where she started, her recovery is still fragile and she still has a long way to go. Addressing the trauma of her daughter's death was incredibly healing, and getting a dog turned out to be a turning point in terms of improving her mood, motivation, and level of physical activity. She will continue connecting with her step daughter's family, which will prove pivotal in her day to day sense of connection and meaning in her life. But she will also struggle with numerous setbacks, including a relapse of smoking after a tree fell on her car during a hurricane. The stress of that, including financial strain, wrangling with the insurance company and needing to get rides to do just about anything left her feeling overwhelmed. The therapist is appalled at the degree to which one disaster can be financially catastrophic to someone with Sandy's means. But Sandy will be able to quit again successfully after a few weeks. Despite her progress with physical activity and a greatly improved diet, she will experience a deep vein thrombosis (DVT) or blood clot in her leg. The blood thinners will cause her to bleed rectally again, and she will feel rather hopeless for a time. "Honestly sometimes I feel like God is just telling me to cash it in," she will say. But the dog, and her relationship with Stephanie and her baby will pull her through. "I guess I still got lots of reasons to keep on kickin'," she will conclude when the therapist encourages her to consider reasons for living, despite her many challenges. Although the Humira will be helpful, her doctor will eventually switch her to Stelara. It will work far better, but she will still ultimately need surgery to correct the fistula. The recovery from the surgery will be painful and slow, but she will be incredibly relieved to not leak stool from her vagina anymore. After about 18 months of work, Sandy will announce one day "Ok doc, I'm ready to graduate. I think you taught me everything I need to know. I'm real grateful, and I want to free up this slot so you can help some other poor slob who needs you more than I do now." The therapist will congratulate Sandy on all her hard work and will remind her of how amazingly resilient, loving, and courageous she is, and how she has built a life of meaning and joy. "Well thanks," Sandy will say. "But I hope you know you helped a little!"

Summary

Chris, Chantal, Julie, Arun, and Sandy are people who are as different from each other as they could be. But they all have an IBD, and each and every one of them benefited enormously from a course of GI informed CBT. If you have not previously done much integrative behavioral health work, you might be surprised by the degree to which the therapist needed to know things about IBD and addressed issues like nutritional deficiencies, diet, and medication choices, and actively consulted with physicians. Hopefully these cases illustrate the importance of doing so. But if you are a reasonably experienced CBT therapist, you probably also saw much in these cases that felt familiar. Relaxation training, deep diaphragmatic breathing, behavioral activation, thought records, cognitive reappraisal, de-catastrophizing, motivational interviewing, imaginal and *in vivo* exposure therapy, behavioral experiments, mindfulness, and trauma focused imaginal rescripting are all tried and true, empirically supported interventions which can be mixed and matched depending on the individual patient's exact presentation and treatment goals. Of course, every patient also benefits from culturally informed and responsive care and from therapists who are aware of and can reflect on intersectionality in their client's identities. GI informed CBT can be literally lifesaving, and can dramatically reduce distress and disability and improve health related quality of life for patients with IBD. It is my hope that these cases will inspire you to take on more of these patients and that this treatment manual will help you feel confident and competent in doing so. It is deeply satisfying work, and we sorely need more therapists who are trained to do it!

Acknowledgments

If it weren't for Dianne Chambless, the field of clinical psychology might still be struggling to figure out what empirically supported treatments are and why they are so important. I was fortunate to count Dianne as a friend and colleague, and there is no question that working with her pushed me to be a better clinical scientist. So here you go Dianne—a treatment manual that blends the best of an EST with the best of flexible deployment of empirically supported principles and transdiagnostic, evidence based interventions and techniques. I hope you would approve. I promise to keep testing it.

This treatment manual reflects the cumulative effort and wisdom of a number of people in the field of gastropsychology, members of the Rome Gastropsych Group, and several wonderful gastroenterologists, including Mark Osterman and C.S. Tse, whom it has been my pleasure to collaborate with over the years. I am grateful to all of them and especially to the Rome group for providing excellent case consultation, resources and support.

My work developing this treatment approach for patients with IBD has benefited from the help of a number of undergraduate research assistants over the years, including Enitan Marcelle, Lauren Rodriguez, Lauren Smith, Paddy Loftus, Michael Accardo, Mary Keenan, Ben Gibbons, Lauren Cohen, Charlotte Gendler, Duy Li, and Elyssia Baskins.

Of course, I could never have done any of this without working with the many patients over the years who have trusted me with their challenges, struggles, and triumphs. I have learned so much about resilience and courage from all of you. Thank you for letting me join you on your journey. I hope working with me has made coping with Crohn's or colitis a little easier.

The pursuit of multicultural competence is a lifelong journey, not a destination or a goal at which one can arrive. I am very grateful to the many people in my life who have been willing to teach and guide me and to call me out and help me grow and learn when I get things wrong. This includes numerous colleagues like Jade Logan, Anu Asnaani, Janeé M. Steele, Jeff Cohen, and Colleen A. Sloan. It also includes my graduate students and interns, especially Kelly Allred, Rivka Cohen and Pankhuri Aggarwal, pretty much all of whom are more aware, informed, thoughtful, and passionate about these issues than just about anyone of my generation. It also includes my adult children, Ian, Noah, and Anna Rose, and my wonderful daughter-in-law, Sudarshana Chanda. Each of them has in turn been brave and gentle, honest and supportive, forthright and kind, and they have all been willing to have tough conversations with me when it was needed. I'm very grateful to all of them for helping me actualize my good intentions. I hope my patients benefit from the tutelage all these wonderful, wise people have given me. That said, my representations of a therapist trying to address intersectionality in the therapeutic relationship are mine alone, and anything that remains clueless or cringy is on me.

A huge thanks to my parents, Robert Hunt and Irene Winter, who are still with me at 89 and 83, and who still provide insightful counsel when I'm working on something and celebratory cheers when it comes to fruition.

And finally, as always, a huge thanks to my beloved husband Garth Isaak, the best partner in work, love, play, parenting, plumbing, and life that I could possibly imagine. If I had to choose what I couldn't lose, it begins and ends with you.

Index

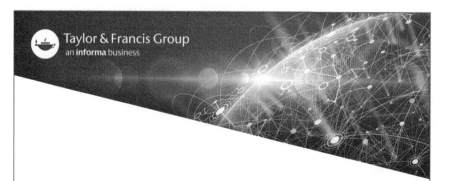